Study Guide

Animal Management

Level 3 Technical - Exam 031/531

The publisher gratefully acknowledges the permission of copyright holders to reproduce copyright material:

p6 (right) Puripatch Lokakalin©123RF.COM, (left) Inna Zakharchenko©123RF.COM

p17 (top left) Juan Gaertner©123RF.COM, (top right) woodoo007©123RF.COM, (middle left) Tatiana Shepeleva©123RF.COM, (middle right) Kateryna Kon©123RF.COM, (bottom left) Pongsak Tawansaeng©123RF.COM

p41, 42 modelling services provided by Poppy

p46 (top left) PENCHAN PUMILA©123RF.COM, (middle right) areeya©123RF.COM, (bottom right) mtsaride©123RF.COM

p66 (right part (c)) Roberto Biasini©123RF.COM

p67 (both) Anton Lebedev©123RF.COM

p72 guniita©123RF.COM

p73 Teguh Mujiono©123RF.COM

p77 designua©123RF.COM

Cover image: Anatolii Tsekhmister©123RF.COM

All other photographs and illustrations are © Eboru Publishing.

Every effort has been made to trace copyright holders and to obtain their permission for the use of copyright material. The publisher will be glad to make arrangements with any copyright holder it has not been possible to contact.

Copyright © 2019 Eboru Publishing

First edition 2019.

ISBN 978-0-9929002-2-9

Ordering Information

Special discounts are available for class set purchases by schools, colleges and others. For details, contact the publisher at: enquiries@eboru.com

Trade orders: copies of this book are available through the normal wholesalers.

For any queries please contact: orders@eboru.com

www.eboru.com

Features in this book

Topic introduction

Brief summary of what you will cover in the next section.

In this topic you will learn about:

- The Animal Welfare Act (2006) and the Animal Health and Welfare Act (Scotland) (2006)

- Welfare of Animals (Transport) Order 2006

- The Welfare of Animals at Market Order 1993

Quiz Questions

Knowledge-check questions at the end of each section, so that you can quickly recap on what you have learned.

Quiz Questions

1 What is the purpose of the Veterinary Surgeon's Act 1966?

2 Name two things that the The Welfare of Animals at Market Order 1993 forbids.

3 According to the Animal Welfare Act 2006, list two things that owners of animals must ensure.

Jargon Buster

There are lots of technical and specialist terms that you will come across whilst studying. This feature will explain what these specialist words mean.

Jargon Buster

Gait the movement of the limbs of as the animal walks or runs

Activity

Tasks that will help you build your knowledge and understanding of the subject.

Activity

For your chosen species, research some of the diseases that occur most commonly that are not listed above.

Contents

Answers to questions are available at www.eboru.com

Unit 303 Animal Health and Husbandry

LO1 Recognise indicators of health in animals

1.1 Signs of health in animals

In this topic you will learn about:

- health indicators in animals, including temperature, pulse rate, respiration rate and capillary refill time

- routine health checks, such as appetite, behaviour, movement and gait, appearance of eyes / ears / nose /mouth / teeth / skin / fur / feathers / scales, appearance of mucous membranes, condition of limbs and feet, faeces and urine, genitals and anal area, coughing / sneezing / vomiting, body condition, weight.

Health indicators

Animals can't tell us when they are feeling ill and so we need to know how to recognise the signs that an animal is ill. You need to know the normal range of readings, and how to measure, the following:

Temperature

It is generally accepted that rectal thermometers provide the most accurate readings. You can use digital thermometers or mercury thermometers. A digital thermometer will make a sound once an accurate temperature has been measured and displays the temperature as a number. When using a mercury thermometer you need to wait for the mercury to stop moving and then read the temperature from the scale.

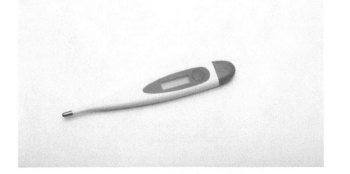

Figure 3.1 A digital thermometer

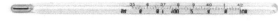

Figure 3.2 A mercury thermometer

To take a temperature reading:

- add lubricant to the measurement probe

- lift the animal's tail and insert the probe into the rectum

- wait until you hear a beep (digital) or until the reading has stabilised (mercury) then read the and record the measurement

- remove the probe, clean and disinfect.

Normal Rectal Temperature Ranges	Temperature in Celcius
Cow	36.7–39.3
Cat	38.1–39.2
Dog	37.9–39.9
Horse	37.2 - 38.3
Pig	38.7–39.8
Rabbit	38.6–40.1
Sheep	38.3–39.9

Adapted from Robertshaw D. Temperature Regulation and Thermal Environment, in Dukes' Physiology of Domestic Animals, 12th ed., Reece WO, Ed. Copyright 2004 by Cornell University.

Pulse Rate

You can take a pulse by locating a major artery and lightly pressing your index and middle finger against it. The best location is different for each animal but some common locations are:

- cattle: underneath the base of the tail

- sheep and goats: at the top of inside back leg

- pigs: at the top of inside back leg

- horse: the jaw/cheek

- dog: at the top of inside back leg

- cat: at the top of inside back leg.

You can count the beats over a full minute, or count over 30 seconds and multiply by two.

Normal pulse rate values	Beats per minute
Cat	120–140
Dairy cow	48–84
Dog	70–120
Hamster	300–600

Horse	28–40
Pig	70–120
Rabbit	180–350
Sheep	70–80

Adapted from Detweiler DK and Erickson HH, Regulation of the Heart, in Dukes' Physiology of Domestic Animals, 12th ed., Reece WO, Ed. Copyright 2004 by Cornell University.

Respiration rate

You can measure respiration – i.e. breathing – by either counting the rise and fall of the animal's chest visually, or you can place your hand on the flank of the animal and count it that way. You need to count the number of breaths over a minute.

Typical respiration rates	Rate per minute
Cat	16–40
Dairy cow	26–50
Dog	18–34
Horse	10–14
Pig	32–58
Sheep	16–34

Adapted from Reece WO, Respiration in Mammals, in Dukes' Physiology of Domestic Animals, 12th ed., Reece WO, Ed. Copyright 2004 by Cornell University.

Capillary refill time (CRT)

A capillary is a very small blood vessel. Capillary refill time (CRT) is how long it takes for blood to return to a section of the capillary system after its supply has been interrupted.

To measure CRT you need to press firmly on the animal's gums (so that part of the gum turns white), then release your finger and time how long it takes for the blood to flow back to that portion of the gum and return to its normal colour. CRT in a healthy animal is normally less than two seconds.

Quiz Questions

1 Name two health indicators in animals.

2 Briefly describe what Capillary Refill Time is.

3 What is considered to be a normal Capillary Refill Time?

4 What is the difference between a digital and mercury thermometer?

Routine health checks

Daily checks

Appetite and water intake
- Record if the animal has eaten a normal amount of food and water since the last time they were fed. Has the animal's appetite changed?

Faeces and urine
- What colour is the urine?
- Is there a change in the consistency of faeces?
- Is the animal passing faeces or urine more or less often than normal?

Behaviour
- Is there a change in the animal's temperament?
- Are they quieter, more timid or more fearful than normal?
- Are they more aggressive than normal?
- Do they appear to be in any pain?

Movement and gait
- Is the animal moving normally?
- Do they appear to have any restrictive movements?
- Does their posture look normal?
- Does their gait look normal – are their limbs co-ordinated, are they staggering, shuffling or missing a stride?

Jargon Buster
gait the movement of the limbs of as the animal walks or runs

Weekly checks

Appearance of eyes, ears, nose, mouth/teeth
- Are the eyes bright, clear and free from cloudiness?
- Are the ears free of any unusual discharge?
- Is the nose free of any unusual discharge? Is the nose in good condition?
- Are the mouth and teeth in good condition? Are they a normal colour? Are there any unusual smells?

Appearance of skin/fur/feathers/scales
- Are the fur, coat, or feathers glossy?
- Are the scales shiny?

- Is the fur matted or in bad condition?

- Are there any visible sores, broken skin or other damage?

- Is there any evidence of lick marks (which is a sign of good health)?

Appearance of mucous membranes

The gums or the tongue are good places to assess the condition of the mucous membrane. The following colours can indicate the following:

- A white mucous membrane may mean the animal is in shock, or has a low count of red blood cells due to bleeding.

- A pink mucous membrane is normal.

- A red mucous membrane can be a sign of an infection or heat stroke.

- A blue mucous membrane is a sign of low oxygen content in the blood.

- A yellow mucous membrane is a sign that there may be a liver or kidney problem.

Appearance of limbs and feet

- Is the animal walking freely or limping?

- Is the animal using all limbs equally?

- Are there any areas of swelling?

- Are the feet or hooves in good condition, without sores or signs of infection?

- Are the claws in good condition, not overly long or twisted out of shape?

Genitals and anal area

- Is there any discharge?

- Are there any unusual smells?

Signs of coughing, sneezing or vomiting

- Is the animal exhibiting any of these?

Monthly check

Body condition

- Does the animal look in good condition?

- Is the animal over or underweight?

- Is the animal rapidly gaining or losing weight?

Your organisation will have procedures in place regarding the monitoring, tracking and reporting of ill-health. You must ensure that

> **Jargon Buster**
> mucous membrane a layer of cells that surrounds certain organs and openings in the body. Such openings include the inner nose, mouth and tongue. The membrane often secretes a fluid, known as mucous. The mucous membrane protects those areas from infection and stops them from drying out.

you are up to date with those procedures and know with whom to discuss any serious or rapid changes in health.

Quiz Questions

1 Name two weekly health checks.

2 What does 'gait' mean?

3 What is a mucous membrane?

4 What do the following mucous membrane colours indicate?
   a   Pink
   b   Blue
   c   Yellow.

1.2 Legislation that relates to animal health

In this topic you will learn about:

- **The Animal Welfare Act (2006) and the Animal Health and Welfare Act (Scotland) (2006)**

- **Welfare of Animals (Transport) Order 2006**

- **The Welfare of Animals at Market Order 1993**

- **The Veterinary Surgeons Act 1966**

- **The Welfare of Farmed Animals Regulations 2007**

- **The Welfare of Animals Regulations 1999 (slaughter or killing)**

- **Horse Passport Regulations 2009 (for those studying Horse Care).**

Animal Welfare Act 2006 and Animal Health and Welfare Act (Scotland) 2006

Aim: To ensure all animals have all of their welfare needs met.

Purpose: To make it illegal for anyone to mistreat animals. Owners or keepers need to ensure that five animal welfare needs are met:

- have a normal diet

- are housed in a suitable environment (place to live)

- are housed with or without other animals, as is considered normal for that particular species

- are free of 'pain, injury, suffering and disease'

- exhibit behaviour that is normal for that species.

Previous to this Act action to tackle animal cruelty could only be taken once the cruelty had taken place. This Act allows authorities to act if it is clear that animals' welfare needs are not being met.

Welfare of Animals (Transport) Order 2006

Aim: To regulate how animals are transported from place to place.

Purpose: To enforce minimum requirements on the transportation of vertebrate animals in line with commercial activities. This means that there are rules about the following:

- whether an animal can be transported in the first place
- how much space different animals must be given
- how long journeys can last for without a break for food and water, e.g. for cattle and sheep any journey over 14 hours requires a one-hour break for watering and feeding
- provision of adequate food and water
- adequate ventilation and temperature
- provision of litter for toileting
- the transporter must be able to provide first aid.

This is not an exhaustive list. The rules are slightly different for different animals, and animal welfare must be checked throughout the journey. If animals are travelling for more than 50km then the vehicle must have an animal transport certificate that includes details about where the animals came from, are going and how long they have been travelling for, amongst other things.

The Welfare of Animals at Market Order 1993

Aim: To cover what happens to animals when they are at markets and shows.

Purpose: To provide some additional responsibilities on the market operator for the welfare of animals at a market, with strict penalties for those who break these rules. In practice this covers things like:

- an animal can't be sold at market if it is pregnant
- animals may not be tied up or suspended off the ground
- the operator must ensure that the animals have enough bedding, food, water, lighting etc.

The Veterinary Surgeons Act 1966

Aim: to regulate vets

Purpose: this Act states that someone can only operate on animals, or call themselves a vet, if they are listed on a register of veterinary surgeons. It states the procedures on animals that non-vets are allowed to perform, and those that only vets can perform. There are some amendments to the Act that were made in 1988 and 2002.

The Welfare of Farmed Animals Regulations 2007

Aim: to implement EU regulations on the welfare of farmed livestock.

Purpose: these regulations are made under the Animal Welfare Act 2006. These regulations have been made to ensure that the Act implements all relevant EU directives on farming animals, which the UK had previously signed up to. The Regulations replace the The Welfare of Farmed Animals (England) 2000 and remove duplication that exists between the 2000 Regulations and the Animal Welfare Act 2006.

The Welfare of Animals Regulations 1999 (slaughter or killing)

Aim: to regulate slaughterhouses

Purpose: to ensure that

- animals are not caused any avoidable pain or suffering
- that the responsibility for the welfare of animals lies with the persons in authority
- that the industry is regulated by requiring licenses for people slaughtering or killing animals.

Horse Passport Regulations 2009

Those studying Horse Care will also need to be aware of these Regulations.

Aim: to keep track of horses that end up in the human food chain.

Purpose: To make it a legal requirement for all horses to be issued with a passport and microchipped. It is an offense for someone to own a horse that does not have a passport. Horses cannot be sold without a passport. The passport is required so that horses that have been administered certain medicines are not slaughtered for humans consumption. This is part of an EU-wide initiative. Whilst horse is not a popular animal to eat in the UK, horses here are slaughtered and sold in certain countries for meat.

Legislation specific to species

Beyond the listed legislation there may be other pieces of legislation that are relevant to the animals or species you are working with. You should make sure you are aware of this legislation. In addition, legislation does change in time, and may be more likely to do so with the UK's departure from the EU. You should make sure you know of any upcoming changes to the list above.

Quiz Questions

1 What is the purpose of the Veterinary Surgeon's Act 1966?

2 Name two things that the The Welfare of Animals at Market Order 1993 forbids.

3 According to the Animal Welfare Act 2006, list two things that owners of animals must ensure.

4 Which institutions does The Welfare of Animals Regulations 1999 (slaughter or killing) regulate?

LO2 Understand common diseases and disorders, their treatment and prevention

2.1 The role of pathogenic organisms in animal disease

In this topic you will learn about:

- *The structure, common types, and replication of pathogenic organisms: bacteria, viruses, fungi, protozoa, parasites.*

- *The lifecycles, symptoms, treatment and prevention of different types of parasites: worms, fleas, ticks, mites, lice.*

Pathogenic organisms

Pathogens are very small organisms – known as microorganisms – that cause disease.

	Bacteria	Virus	Fungi	Protozoa	Parasite
Structure	Single-celled organisms that belong to class of cells called prokaryotes – they have a cell wall but do not have a membrane-bound nucleus or contain mitochondria. (Animal and plant cells belong to a class of cells called eukaryotes). Bacteria are neither plants nor animals.	Simple organisms that consist of genetic material, either DNA or RNA, surrounded by a protective protein 'coat'. They are non-living organisms as they require a host cell in order to reproduce.	Multicellular fungi are made up of fungal cells that are organised into thread-like structures called hyphae. Single cell fungi, such as yeast, are not organised into hyphae.	Single-celled organisms that display animal-like characteristics, such as movement and feeding.	A parasite is any organism that lives on another organism. Pathogenic parasites in animals tend to either be protozoa, ticks or worms.

	Bacteria	Virus	Fungi	Protozoa	Parasite
Size	Measured in micrometres, which are a millionth of a metre i.e. a thousand times smaller than a millimetre!	Measured in nanometres, which are a thousand-millionth of a metre – or a million times smaller than a millimetre. This means that the smallest viruses are a thousand times smaller than typical bacteria.	Varies enormously – from microscopic to very large indeed.	Microscopic	Parasites vary in size.

	Bacteria	Virus	Fungi	Protozoa	Parasite
Replication	Bacteria replicate asexually in a process known as binary fission. When a cell is big enough it replicates its genetic material and then divides into two, with each cell containing the same genetic material. Genetic material can be transferred between different bacterial cells through a different process known as conjugation (which facilitates bacterial resistance to antibiotics).	They are so small that they can get into cells; once there they reproduce themselves by taking over the cell's normal reproduction process.	Fungi can reproduce sexually or asexually. Sexual reproduction occurs when two parent cells of opposite strains fuse, which leads to new cells that are genetically different to the parent. In asexual reproduction the fungus develops spores which are genetically identical to the parent cells. The spores are then dispersed, and then grow into new hyphae. Yeasts reproduce asexually by budding.	Protozoa can reproduce sexually or asexually. The most common asexual reproduction is binary fission, as per bacteria. However other asexual reproductiuon includes budding and plasmotomy.	Fleas, ticks, mites, lice and worms reproduce by laying eggs inside their host.

	Bacteria	Virus	Fungi	Protozoa	Parasite
Examples of common types	E. coli, staphylococcus, salmonella (salmonella), Staphylococcus aureus, Streptococcus pneumoniae (pneumonia), Bacillus anthracis (anthrax).	Foot and Mouth disease, influenza strains.	Candida (a yeast, responsible for thrush), tinea (ringworm athlete's foot and other skin infections), mushrooms.	Plasmodium (responsible for malaria), amoeba, Trypanosoma brucei (responsible for African sleeping sickness), Toxoplasma gondii.	See next section for examples.

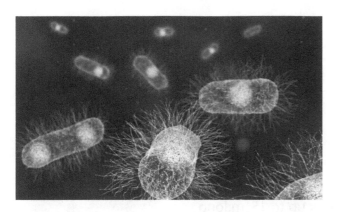

Figure 3.3 Bacteria

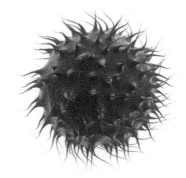

Figure 3.4 Virus

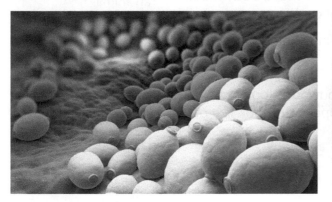

Figure 3.5 Fungus

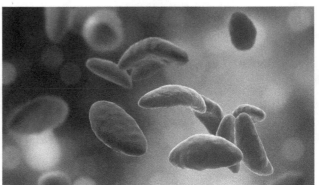

Figure 3.6 Protozoa

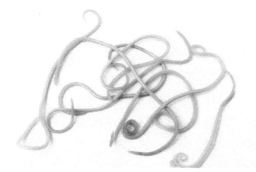

Figure 3.7 The intestinal worm is a parasite

Quiz Questions

1 What is the structure of bacteria?

2 How does a virus replicate?

3 What is a protozoa?

4 List the names of two common types of bacteria.

5 For each of the diseases listed in Section 2.2 state whether they are caused by bacteria, viruses, fungi, protozoa or parasites.

Parasites

Parasites get their food from their host. Endoparasites live in an animal, e.g. worms. Ectoparasites live on an animal, e.g. fleas, ticks, mites, lice.

Worms

Worms are invertebrate organisms that can live within an animal's body. There are two main types of worm:

- roundworms – these are round, white, and grow up to 15cm long

- tapeworms – these are flat, consisting of a head with a body made of independent segments, and grow up to 60cm long

Both of these normally live in the animal's small intestine.

Symptoms of worms are:

- presence of worms in faeces or vomit – roundworms look like small white pieces of string, whilst fragments of tapeworms look like or small grains of rice

- diarrhoea

- anaemia

- dehydration

- loss of weight

- pot belly

- behaviour indicating an itching anus.

However these may only appear when the infestation is advanced. Prior to that there may not be any obvious symptoms.

The lifecycle of a roundworm is as follows:

- Eggs are laid in the intestine and pass out of the body with the animal's droppings or vomit.

- Larvae develop after about two weeks whilst still in the eggshell. The

> **Jargon Buster**
>
> invertebrate an organism without a backbone
>
> parasites organisms who obtain food from another host organism
>
> endoparasites live in an animal
>
> ectoparasites live on an animal

eggs are sticky and will attach to animals' fur and then be ingested when the animal cleans itself.

- Once inside an animal's stomach, the egg hatches and this second stage larvae makes its way to the small intestine and from there, the liver.

- Third stage larvae develops in the liver, which then move through blood vessels into the heart and then lungs. The animal will cough the larvae up and swallow it.

- The larvae makes its way via the stomach to the small intestine, where it reaches adulthood and begins to lay more eggs.

The total lifecycle is about six weeks. If the animal is pregnant then the roundworm can infect the unborn animal. It is not uncommon for young puppies to already have roundworms and hence puppies and kittens need worming. Common roundworms in the UK are Toxocara canis, which affects dogs, Toxocara cati, which affects cats, and Toxascaris leonina, which affects both.

Unlike roundworms, tapeworms require an intermediate host. **The lifecycle of a tapeworm** is as follows:

- Segments of the tapeworm separate from the main body and pass out of the animal's body. Each segment contains eggs.

- The eggs are then ingested by other organisms. In 'flea tapeworms', flea larvae consume the eggs, which develop into cysts, and can then be carried into an animal if it swallows the flea (perhaps due to biting at an itch due to a fleabite). The ingested tapeworm grows to adulthood in the animal's intestine.

- Other tapeworms, known as 'hydatid tapeworms', can be ingested by other animals, and if they do the eggs develop into cysts in the second animal's organs (offal). If another animal is fed this infected offal, the tapeworm cysts will develop into adults in this third animal.

Common tapeworms in the UK are Dipylidium caninum, various species of Taenia which require an intermediate host, and Echinococcus granulosa, which is a zoonotic disease i.e. can be passed on to humans.

As well as roundworms and tapeworms there are other species of worm that can affect animals in the UK:

- Hookworms resemble roundworms but have teeth that they use to grip the small intenstine.

- Whipworms have a thick end and a thin end, resembling a whip, and live in the large intestine.

- Lungworms are carried by snails and slugs and can infect dogs and cats when eaten. They live in the animal's heart and blood vessels that supply the lungs. Symptoms are breathlessness and coughing. Lungworms are becoming more common in the UK.

- Liver flukes are a type of flatworm and parasite of the liver that affect all mammals but are prevalent in sheep and is a cause of death.

Treatment of worms is normally through de-worming medication – either tablets, injections or spots on the collar. Puppies and kittens need worming as it is quite common for them to become infected by their mothers when in the womb.

Prevention of worms: keep animals free from fleas, dispose of faeces promptly, restrict animals' movement outdoors in order to avoid areas with droppings.

Fleas

Fleas live on the skin and feed off the animal's blood. **Symptoms are**:

- skin irritation
- other allergic reactions
- blood infections.

Evidence for fleas is flea 'dirt' – digested blood excreted by adult fleas, which can be seen by combing the animal's coat onto white paper and looking for dark red or brown specs.

Fleas can also carry other pathogenic organisms which cause more serious problems. For instance fleas carry the deadly rabbit disease myxmatosis.

The lifecycle of a flea is as follows:

- Egg stage: hatches in 2-14 days.
- Larvae stage: lasts 4-20 days. The larvae are blind and feed on pre-digested blood passed from adult fleas. At the end of this stage the larvae spins a cocoon.
- Cocoon or pupae stage: normally lasts a few days to a few weeks, but can last for much longer if the conditions are not right. The cocoon protects the flea in this final development stage.
- Adult fleas emerge from the pupae when it senses that there is a host. Adult fleas live for 2-3 months but can last for much longer in favourable conditions.

Treatment of fleas: there are a few methods to treat fleas - sprays, powders, tablets and shampoos are all available to treat the animal. However a large percentage of the flea population consists of eggs, larvae and pupae. Therefore it is advisable to vacuum, clean and treat the environment as well.

Prevention (or prophylaxis**) of fleas** is normally using tablets, collars, shampoos and sprays that contain ingredients that are toxic for fleas.

Jargon Buster
prophylaxis another word for prevention

Ticks

Ticks move from one host to another and feed off each of the host's blood.

Symptoms are:

- itching and skin irritation

- loss of fur

- dull coat.

Ticks can carry diseases which they pass to the host, including Lyme disease, whose symptoms include lameness or seemingly arthritic joints.

The lifecycle of ticks normally consists of four life stages, with different hosts required at each stage:

- Egg: hatches in a few weeks.

- Larvae: the larvae need to find a host to feed on. If they find one then they take several weeks or longer to develop into nymphs.

- Nymphs: they require another host on which to feed and, again, if they find one they then it takes several weeks to months develop into adults.

- Adults: once the adults have had enough food from their host they will mate and die.

The overall timeframes for each stage can vary enormously because ticks rely on finding a host in order to feed and progress onto the next stage. However if they can't find a host, they can survive without food for a long time. So the overall life of a tick can be measured in years.

Treatment of ticks:

- As with fleas, there are a range of sprays, powders, tablets, collars and shampoos available.

- If a tick is found on an animal it can be removed using specialist equipment. However it is important that ticks are not pulled out as they can leave their mouths embedded in the animal and cause further infection.

Prevention of ticks can be as simple as keeping an animal indoors or restricting their movement when outside. Higher-risk environments include wooded and vegetated areas.

Mites

Mites are similar to ticks but tend to be smaller. They either feed on organic material, like dead skin, or the host's blood. They either live on the surface of the skin or burrow just underneath. It is less common for mites to carry diseases.

Symptoms are:

- itchiness

- sore, dry skin

- dark crusts of skin in the ears can indicate the presence of ear mites

- poor condition, caused by the skin disease mange.

The life cycle for mites is much the same as for ticks:

- eggs

- larvae hatch from the eggs, with three legs
- nymph
- adult, with four legs.

The lifecycle of a mite varies across species but is around 2-4 weeks.

Treatment of mites: chemicals that kill mites and ticks are called acaricides and are available in sprays, dips, shampoos etc.

Prevention of mites: keeping bedding and the environment clean will help to prevent mites but separating infected and non-infected animals is key.

Jargon Buster
acaricides a chemical that kills mites and ticks

Lice

Lice are under 8mm long and are split into 'bloodsucking' and 'biting'. The lice can only live on one species, meaning that lice cannot spread from one species to another.

Symptoms are:

- itching
- bad skin condition
- loss of hair or fur.

The lifecycle for lice all take place on the host:

- eggs are laid in the animal's hair or fur – these eggs are often known as 'nits'
- nymphs hatch from the eggs, and then moult three times, before becoming adults, taking around 10-20 days
- the adults live for another 2-3 weeks.

Treatment of lice: shampoos, powders, sprays are all available to treat the animal and its environment.

Prevention of lice: lice can only survive on the host, and rely on host-to-host contact to spread. So, preventing lice can be as simple as ensuring that animals are closely checked before coming into contact with clean animals, and equipment such as combs and bedding are not shared with infected or unchecked animals.

Quiz Questions

1. What is the definition of a parasite?

2. What is an endoparasite?

3. Describe the lifecycle of a tapeworm.

4. What are the symptoms of dog that has ticks?

5. How should you treat a cat with fleas?

Methods of disease transmission

Diseases are spread through the transmission of pathogens. Pathogens can be spread in different ways:

- Direct transmission: This is when animals come into physical contact with each other, either by touching directly or via bodily fluids. Pathogens that require direct contact to transmit do not survive for long in the environment away from a host, and are easy to kill.

- Indirect: Some pathogens can survive for a long time in the environment, away from a host. Because of this they are harder to kill.

- Airborne: some pathogens can remain suspended in the air e.g. after coughing or sneezing.

- Pathogens normally need to get inside an animal to cause it problems.

- Inhalation: requires the animal to breathe in a pathogen which is airborne.

- Ingestion: diseases transmitted through eating or drinking.

- Other entry points: pathogens can also enter directly into the bloodstream through cuts or grazes, or through biting parasites.

Indirect transmission occurs in one of two ways:

- Fomite: any non-living object that can contain and transmit diseases e.g. bedding, food containers. Pathogens transmitted this way are picked up through the animal's environment.

- Vectors: some pathogens are spread by other organisms – these organisms are called vectors of the disease. E.g. the tick Ixodes ricinus is the principal vector for Lyme disease. Vectors can be split into mechanical, where the pathogen is simply carried by the vector, and biological – where the pathogen requires the vector as part of its lifecycle.

Immunity

All animals have an immune system of antibodies that helps to protect them against diseases. This system can identify pathogens that have entered the animal's body and kill them.

- Natural immunity: an animal will already have immunity to a range of diseases. This will vary across species and individual animals within the species.

- Passive immunity: this is when an animal is given another animal's antibodies which can fight off disease. This commonly happens between a mother and offspring through feeding with colostrum, which is the initial form of milk developed by a mammalian mother. Passive immunity is only acquired if colostrum is consumed by a newborn within a day of birth.

- Active immunity: an animal may become infected by a pathogen and develop a disease, but their immune system will still try to produce antibodies to kill the pathogen. If the animal recovers from the disease then its immune system is likely to have learned to create the correct antibodies. For some diseases this means that the animal has become immune to the disease and will not catch it again.

- Artificial immunity: because the immune system can be trained to produce antibodies, injecting a small amount of a pathogen into animal – known as a vaccine – can ensure that the animal becomes immune to the disease. (This is also the basis of jabs given to humans at various stages in their life.)

In the case of active and artificial immunity special types of white blood cells, called B-cell and T-cells, are able to recognise new pathogens, react to them and then 'remember' the chemical structure of the disease, in order that the body can generate the same response if the pathogen is detected again in the future.

Symptoms of disease

Some common diseases and their symptoms are given in section 2.2.

In some cases an animal, or human, can carry a pathogen but not contract the disease. However they can still transmit the pathogen to other animals who may contract the disease. These are known as asymptomatic carriers.

> **Jargon Buster**
> antibodies proteins that are produced in the blood in response to pathogens detected in the body, that are able to kill pathogens.
>
> vaccine a small and specially controlled amount of pathogen introduced into a body specifically to stimulate the production of antibodies that can fight off the pathogen
>
> asymptomatic carrier an animal that carries a disease but does not contract it themselves

Quiz Questions

1 List three methods of disease transmission.

2 What is a fomite?

3 What is a vector?

4 What is an antibody?

5 Describe how artificial immunity works.

6 Explain what an asymptomatic carrier is.

2.2 Common diseases and disorders in animals and their impact on health and welfare

In this topic you will learn about the signs and symptoms, treatment and prevention of the following:

- Notifiable diseases: rabies, avian flu, swine flu, BSE, tuberculosis, bluetongue. foot and mouth disease, Newcastle disease, equine infectious anaemia;

- Zoonotic diseases: ringworm, salmonella, campylobacter, cat scratch fever, leptospirosis, Lyme disease, psittacosis, cheyletiella, sarcoptic mange, toxoplasmosis.

Notifiable diseases

A notifiable disease means that there is a legal requirement to report them to the Animal and Plant Health Agency. This includes any suspicion that an animal has the disease, even if you are not sure.

Notifiable disease	Signs and symptoms	Treatment	Prevention and control
Rabies – a virus that attacks the nervous system, spread through bites from infected animals.	Behavioural change, aggression, sensitivity to light, fever, paralysis of the jaw, foaming at the mouth.	Once the disease develops there is no cure.	Vaccinations against rabies are the most effective prevention. In the UK there is a vaccination programme in place for cats, dogs and ferrets. Domesticated animals should avoid wild or rabid animals. In the UK there are pet travel rules that control the movement of animals crossing the border. Companion animals that do not follow the pet travel rules are put into quarantine for 4 months upon entry into the UK. As there is no cure, animals that are suspected of the having the disease in the UK are quarantined for observation. If they do not recover from symptoms or it is otherwise confirmed they have the disease, they will be put down.

Notifiable disease	Signs and symptoms	Treatment	Prevention and control
Avian flu – also known as 'bird flu', this virus is transmitted by direct contact between birds or through bodily fluids and faeces. It is not an airborne disease.	Swollen head, breathing problems, coughing, sneezing, blue tinge to head, diarrhoea, reduced appetite, fewer laid eggs.	There are two versions of avian flu – birds with the low pathogenicity version will normally get better by themselves but the high pathogenicity version is deadly and there is currently no known cure.	Vaccines have been developed but their effectiveness is uncertain. Avian flu is highly infectious so the best prevention is to prevent contact with infected birds, particularly wild birds. Any birds with symptoms should be isolated immediately, and the area cleaned and disinfected.
Swine flu – a virus that spreads between pigs through direct contact and airborne transmission – much like human flu.	Breathing difficulties, coughing, sneezing, reduced appetite, weight loss.	Swine flu is rarely fatal in pigs, so treatment is limited to rest and recuperation for infected pigs.	Vaccines are available but are not always effective because the virus regularly mutates into new strains. Preventing contact between healthy and infected pigs is the best prevention strategy, alongside cleaning and disinfecting areas where infected pigs have been.
Bovine Spongiform Encephalopathy (BSE) – also known as 'mad cow disease' is a very serious disease which affects the central nervous system of cattle and is due to problems with a specific protein.	Loss of muscle control, problems with balance and coordination, mood or behavioural changes. It has a long incubation period which means that infected cows may not display symptoms for years.	There is currently no known cure for BSE.	BSE is caused by cows being fed infected cows or sheep in the form of meat and bone meal (MBM). Thus the main prevention measure has been an ban on feeding MBM to cattle. In addition there are strict rules about disposal of carcasses in slaughterhouses – e.g. brain and spinal cords are categorised as Specified Risk Material (SRM) and are removed in abattoirs before any meat processing.

Notifiable disease	Signs and symptoms	Treatment	Prevention and control
Tuberculosis – a bacterial disease that normally produces nodules in the lungs of mammals and birds. Transmission is airborne, due to coughing or sneezing. If untreated in can lead to death	Symptoms take some time to develop but include loss of appetite, fever, coughing, diarrhoea and prominent lymph nodes.	Animals are rarely treated for the disease.	Prevention is normally simply through slaughter of infected animals. Vaccines have also been developed but are not as widespread or effective as human vaccines. In high risk areas cattle are tested for the disease every four years.
Bluetongue – a viral disease, transmitted through midge bites, that is most common in sheep.	Fever, swollen face, nasal discharge and salivation, foot lesions, blue tongue (though not always)	There is no treatment available – the focus is on prevention.	Vaccination, quarantine of infected animal and control of the midge, which is a vector for the disease.
Foot and mouth disease – infectious viral disease, affecting cattle, sheep, goats, pigs and other cloven-hoofed animals. The virus is spread by direct contact, through airborne tranmission or by fomites. The disease is rarely fatal.	Fever, blisters in the mouth, excessive salivation and drooling, blistering on the feet.	There is no treatment.	Vaccinations (not always effective as the virus continually evolves). Quarantine and disinfection are applied to affected farms, and eventually infected animals are culled, as well as those in a zone near to the outbreak. The last major outbreak of Foot and Mouth in the UK was in 2001.
Newcastle disease- an infectious viral disease affecting birds, spread through direct contact with infected birds and their bodily fluids, and also through fomites. It can lead to death in acute cases.	Breathing difficulties, coughing, depressed appearance, twisted head/neck, reduced egg production.	There is no treatment available.	Vaccination and isolation of infected animals.

Notifiable disease	Signs and symptoms	Treatment	Prevention and control
Equine Infectious Anaemia - a viral disease affecting horses, transmitted by blood, with biting horseflies acting as vectors. However it can also be passed on through shared syringes when administering vaccines or treatment. Female horses can also pass to unborn foals. The acute form will lead to death.	Fever, tiredness, loss of appetite, weight loss, weakness, depressed behaviour, and anaemia	There is no treatment available.	Use disposable needles, limit contact with wild animals, and isolate immediately if symptoms are displayed. Infected animals are often destroyed in order to prevent further spread of the disease.

Zoonotic diseases

A zoonotic disease is an infectious disease that can be passed on to humans. When handling animals that have, or are suspected of having a zoonotic disease, special measures must be put in place:

- Handlers must wear appropriate personal protective equipment (PPE).

- Infecton control practices must be in place to prevent the spread of the disease – this is sometimes known as barrier nursing.

- Other biosecurity measures include: isolation rooms for infected animals that can be easily cleaned and disinfected; limited access to these rooms e.g. with a sign-in sheet; minimum number of people to have contact with animals; dedicated equipment only for use with infected animals; dispoable equipment/clothing; complete separation of non-infected and infected animals.

Zoonotic disease	Signs and symptoms	Treatment	Prevention and control
Ringworm – not a worm but a fungus which lives in the top layer of the skin and in hair follicles, and is spread through direct contact. It is not life-threatening.	Circular patches (which give the disease its name), red and scabby skin, patches of hair or fur loss, dry and brittle coat, brittle claws.	Topical treatments (creams, shampoo, ointments) and anti-fungal oral medication. Cleaning and treatment of the animal's environment to remove infected hair.	Keeping the environment clean is the main preventative measure. Vaccines are available e.g. Ringvac.

Zoonotic disease	Signs and symptoms	Treatment	Prevention and control
Salmonella – a bacterial infection of the intestine that many animals carry without becoming ill. The bacteria can be passed on to unborn animals from their mother, or by direct contact. The bacteria are present in faeces and can then contaminate the environment. In addition it can be spread through eating contaminated meat or animal products.	Many animals naturally have the bacteria and are not ill. But animals that do get ill have symptoms such as diarrhoea, vomiting, fever and loss of appetite.	Antibiotics, and ensuring the animal is sufficiently hydrated.	Keeping animals' living areas clean, and cleaning up animal faeces, will help prevent transmission between animals. Humans should thoroughly wash their hands after touching animals to avoid contracting the disease.
Campylobacter – a bacterial infection that lives in the gut. Like Salmonella, many animals have the bacteria but do not get ill; and the bacteria is spread in much the same way. The bacteria is particularly common in poultry but they rarely contract the disease.	For the animals that do get sick, symptoms include fever, diarrhoea, lack of appetite, vomiting.	Antibiotics are available for acute cases involving pets.	Vaccination and keeping animal living areas clean, control of animal faeces to prevent contamination of water supplies, Most human cases are due to handling raw poultry or undercooking it.
Cat Scratch Fever – a bacterial infection carried by cats but they rarely get ill. It spreads between cats through a flea vector. It can however affect other animals.	Fever, swelling of lymph nodes, coughing, lesions on the skin, weight loss, tiredness.	Antibiotics.	Prevention of fleas and ticks.

Zoonotic disease	Signs and symptoms	Treatment	Prevention and control
Leptospirosis – a bacterial disease spread through the urine of animals, often passed on through contaminated water.	Vomiting, fever, abdominal pain, diarrhea, weakness, loss of appetite.	Antibiotics.	Rodents such as rats and mice are often responsible for infection, so limiting exposure to them help prevent the disease. Vaccinations are also available though are not always 100% effective.
Lyme Disease – a bacterial disease transmitted by a tick vector. It is not transmitted directly from animal to animal.	Fever, swelling of joints, loss of appetite, lameness.	Antibiotics.	Avoid wild areas where the ticks are found – woods, marshes, tall grasses – and clear overgrown vegetation near animal enclosures. Use tick prevention measures. Vaccinations are also available.
Psittacosis – caused by a bacteria this disease is also known as 'Parrot Fever'. However it can occur in a number of different animals, with different symptoms. Spread through droppings or other bodily secretions.	In birds, eye discharge, breathing problems, diarrhoea, loss of appetite, lethargy.	Antibiotics are available but with mixed results due to the nature of the organism.	Disinfection and cleanliness. Avoidance of wild birds.
Cheyletiella – mites that live on the surface of the skin that look like dandruff. More common on dogs, cats and rabbits.	White flakes in the coat, itching, loss of hair or fur	The usual topical treatments for removing mites – medicated sprays, medicated shampoos, medicated dips etc.	Normally spread through close contact of infected animals, so prevent contact with infected animals.

Zoonotic disease	Signs and symptoms	Treatment	Prevention and control
Sarcoptic mange – a disease of the skin caused by a mite that burrows through the skin. Spread through direct contact or via fomites.	Itching, loss of hair or fur, skin rash, red lesions	Topical treatment (medicated shampoos, medicated dips) for the mites with an antibiotic oral treatment for infections due to damaged skin. Treatments kill the mites but not the eggs, so repeat treatments are necessary.	As with Cheyletiella, spread through close contact of animals, so infected animals should be quarantined and all areas washed and disinfected.
Toxoplasmosis – a parasite found in most mammals but cats are a host for its lifecycle, which means it can only lay eggs in a cat. Cat faeces, and the environment in which they are deposited, are infectious, to cats, other animals and humans. The disease causes pregnant sheep and goats to abort.	Most cats will not show any symptoms of infection. However their faeces and the soil etc. where they are buried are dangerous for pregnant sheep and goats. Pregnant women are also at risk as the parasite can harm unborn children. For this reason pregnant women should avoid contact with sheep during lambing season.	Antibiotics are available for cats who are affected by the disease.	No vaccine is available. Toxoplasmosis carries a significant risk to the unborn child of pregnant women.

Beyond the lists of notifiable and zoonotic diseases given, there are other diseases that are specific to each species. You must ensure that you are familiar with common diseases for your chosen species that are not listed above. For each one you must know about their:

- signs and symptoms
- treatment
- control.

Any animal with symptoms of a disease may be in pain or discomfort and may therefore act aggressively whilst being treated, even if this is completely out of character.

Jargon Buster
notifiable disease a disease which must be reported to the APHA

zoonotic disease a disease which can be passed from animals to humans

Activity

For your chosen species, research some of the diseases that occur most commonly that were not listed previously. In each case find out about their symptoms, treatment and control.

Quiz Questions

1 What is a notifiable disease?

2 What is a zoonotic disease?

3 How should you treat lymes disease?

4 Name two ways you could help prevent an animal contracting lymes disease?

5 What are two symptoms of rabies?

6 How is BSE spread?

7 What kind of animals does Newcastle disease affect?

8 What is sarcoptic mange and how does it spread?

2.3 Reasons and methods of preventative care and treatment measures used for animals

In this topic you will learn about common types and frequency of vaccinations for:

• dogs

• cats

• rabbits

• horses

The advice below is general, as vaccines are constantly being developed and manufacturers have specific usage guidelines. Ensure you are familiar with the advice of the product you use. Some of the diseases below may be treated in combined vaccination programmes.

Dogs

Core vaccinations	Puppy vaccination	Booster
Canine Distemper Virus (CDV)	From 6-12 weeks old, doses every 2-4 weeks until 16 weeks	First booster at 6-12 months, subsequent boosters every 3 years
Canine Parvovirus (CPV)	6-12 weeks old	1-3 years
Canine Adenovirus (CAV)	6-12 weeks old	1-3 years
Non-core vaccinations		
Canine Lepotspira	Two doses, 2-4 weeks apart	1 year
Canine parainfluenza virus	Three doses, every 3-4 weeks once 6-8 weeks old	1-3 years
Bordetella bronchiseptica	Two doses	Annual
Rabies		Only normally required if travelling abroad.

Cat

	Kitten vaccination	Booster
Feline Infectious Enteritis/ Feline Panleucopaenia/Feline Parvovirus	There is a combined course of two vaccinations, at 9 and 12 weeks old, that cover Feline Infectious Enteritis, Feline Herpes and Feline Calicivirus.	Annual.
Feline Herpes	See above.	
Feline Calicivirus	See above.	
Feline Leukaemia Virus	Non-core vaccination. Two initial vaccines, a few weeks apart.	Annual.
Feline Chlamydophilosis	Non-core vaccination, only given to higher risk cases.	
Rabies		Only normally required if travelling abroad.

Rabbit

	First vaccinations	Booster
Myxomatosis / Rabbit Haemorrhagic Disease	This is a combined vaccination for both diseases – given after 5 weeks old.	Annual.
RHD 2 (a new strain of Rabbit Haemorrhagic Disease)	2 weeks later than the vaccine above.	Every 6-12months.

Horse

	First vaccinations	Booster
Tetanus	Two vaccinations: 1st normally given to horses over 5 months old, 2nd given 1-3 months later	Every two years.
Equine influenza	Three vaccinations, with 5 weeks between 1st and 2nd, 6 months between 2nd and 3rd.	Annual.
Equine herpes virus	Two vaccinations: 1st normally given to horses over 5 months old, 2nd 4-6 weeks later.	Every 6 months.
Strangles/*Streptococcus equi.*	Two to three vaccinations every 2-4 weeks	Every 3-6 months.
Equine viral arteritis	For breeding stallions, two vaccinations three weeks apart.	3 weeks before breeding.

Quiz Questions

1 Name a core vaccination for a puppy and state when the vaccinations are made. (You do not need to include the booster)

2 Name a core vaccination for a kitten and state when the vaccinations are made. (You do not need to include the booster)

3 Name an important vaccination for rabbits and state when the vaccinations are made. (You do not need to include the booster.)

4 Name three vaccinations given to horses.

2.4 Causes, signs and treatment of animal nutritional deficiencies, excesses and disorders

In this topic you will learn about: the causes, signs and treatment of common nutritional disorders relevant to a range of species, which includes:

- anorexia

- obesity

- vitamin and mineral deficiency and excess

- protein deficiency

- constipation

- diabetes

- urolithiasis

- laminitis

- equine metabolic syndrome.

	Causes	Signs	Treatment
Anorexia – a loss of appetite	There are many conditions associated with a lack of appetite – see page 25. Could also be caused by change in type of food, environment, weather (e.g. hot summer), some problems with the mouth, throat or teeth.	Animal is not interested in food or does not eat as much as normal.	Look for other symptoms to diagnose the problem.
Obesity – excess weight	Too much food, too little exercise, or both.	Very tired or slow after moderate exercise, visible excess fat around the stomach and rib cage.	Increase exercise and examine the amount and type of food being fed, including treats.

Vitamin deficiency	Causes	Signs	Treatment
Vitamin A	Found in green plants, liver, dairy – so lack of these foods in diet.	Night blindness, problems with reproduction, bad condition of hair and skin.	Correct diet.
Vitamin D	Lack of sun and/or dietary sources, such as fish, grains and hay.	Rickets (weak and curved bones), growth problems, weak legs, soft eggs laid by birds	Exposure to sun and correct diet.
Vitamin E	Lack of fish, oils, cereals, liver, green plants.	Muscular dystrophy, low fertility.	Correct diet.
Vitamin K	Lack of green plants, alfalfa, liver, fish.	Affects ability of blood to clot.	Correct diet.
B1 – Thiamine	Lack of grains, liver.	Anorexia, poor coordination, weakness, convulsions.	Correct diet.
B2 - Riboflavin	Lack of green plants, fungi, cow or goat milk. Ruminants can make their own.	Anorexia, weight loss, skin and eye lesions.	Correct diet.
B6	Lack of liver, vegetables, whole-grain cereals, nuts. However most food contains B6.	Growth problems, skin problems, anaemia, hair or fur loss, convulsions.	Correct diet.
B12	Meat, kidney, liver, dairy, fish. Ruminants can make their own but require cobalt to do so.	Growth problems, anaemia, loss of appetite.	For ruminants, cobalt in the diet. For other animals, correct diet.
Biotin	Present in most food but low in corn, barley, wheat, oats, meat and fish	Hair or fur loss, dermatitis and diarrhoea.	Correct diet
Folic Acid	Beans, nuts, citrus, green plants and meat. Ruminants can make some of their own.	Anaemia, growth problems.	Correct diet and avoidance of folic acid inhibitors.
B3 - Niacin	Most animals can make their own but cats cannot make enough and need dietary sources. Sources include pulses, meat and organs.	Dermatitis, diarrhoea, oral ulcers	For cats, the correct diet.
Vitamin C	Primates and guinea pigs cannot make their own Vitamin C and need dietary sources. Other animals can and are rarely deficient..	Scurvy, fatigue, weakness.	Correct diet for animals that need it.

Mineral deficiency	Causes	Signs	Treatment
Calcium	Key to the formation of strong bones and teeth.	Problems with the skeleton and teeth; resposnible for 'milk fever' (hypocalcaemia) in cattle and sheep, which can lead to coma and death. An animal with early stages of milk fever cannot stand properly (recumbent).	Bone meal and meat.
Phosphorus	In collaboration with calcium, is essential to the formation of strong bones and teeth.	Problems with the skeleton and teeth. Metabolic bone disorder in exotic animals is linked to low phosphorus/calcium/vitamin D.	Found in dairy, vegetables, meat, cereals.
Potassium	Prolonged diarrhoea or vomiting can lead to deficiencies.	Paralysis, loss of muscle mass, urinating frequently, thirst.	Found in dairy, fish, meat, vegetables.
Sodium	Prolonged diarrhoea or vomiting can lead to deficiencies.	Increased heart rate, thirst.	Widely available in normal food sources. Salt is a major source.
Magnesium	Illness or diarrhoea can lead to low levels of magnesium in the blood.	Problems with joints, muscle weakness, paralysis. Causes 'grass staggers' (hypomagnesaemia) in cattle and sheep – they are unable to stand properly, appear over-alert, excitable or aggressive; can lead to convulsions and death.	Available in meat and bone meal, cereals
Iron	Blood loss from wounds or blood-sucking parasites	Anaemia, blood loss, growth problems.	Found in meat. liver and fish.
Zinc	High calcium diet can suppress zinc absorption, as can plant-rich diet. Certain breeds of dog such as Huskies and Malamutes have problems absorbing zinc.	Lesions and bad skin condition, dull coat.	Red meat, fish, cereals and grains.
Copper	More likely to affect sheep and cattle - low level of copper in plants that animals feed on, excessive molybdenum and sulphur in plants/soil.	Hind leg weakness (swayback) in lambs, loss of pigment in hair.	Mineral supplements, copper-rich fertiliser.
Iodine	Low levels of iodine in soil in which crops are grown.	Enlarged thyroid gland, reduced growth, weakness.	Fish is a good source.
Selenium (also linked to Vitamin E)	Rare in cats and dogs, more common in sheep and cattle who graze on selenium-deficient soil	Anorexia, muscular dystrophy.	Treat soil with selelnium-rich fertiliser. Dietary sources are meat, fish, bread.

Protein deficiency	Proteins are made of amino acids; different animals can make different amino acids. Taurine is an amino acid that cats cannot make (synthesise) and needs to be in their diet.	Impaired vision, tooth decay	Found in meat, fish, eggs.
Arachidonic acid	An essential fatty acid that cats cannot make.	Poor skin, vision problems, reproductive issues, problems with blood clotting.	Found in meat.
Constipation	Not the correct amount of fibre, eating non-organic material (e.g. stones), blockage in the colon or anal passage, some medications dehydrate.	Straining, crouching, lack of stools.	Medication (laxatives), treatment of blockages, access to adequate water supplies.
Diabetes	Diabetes normally refers to the condition 'diabetes mellitius', which is when insulin cannot be produced in sufficient quantities, or the body responds inadequately to it. Insulin is critical to the conversion of food into energy. (There is another condition called diabetes insipidus which has similar symptoms but which has a completely different cause. We will not discuss further other than to say It is rare and caused by problems with a hormone that causes the body to produce too much urine.)	Frequently urinating, thirsty, hungry, weight-loss, inactive, dull coat.	Regular exercise helps prevent diabetes. If the condition has developed then insulin injections will be required.
Urolithiasis	Also known as urinary stones, these are caused by a build up of solids in the urinary tract.	Blood in urine, pain when urinating, frequent urination, straining.	Invasive surgery, non-invasive surgery (ultrasound), diet changes, medicine.
Laminitis	Affecting horses and donkeys, this is an inflammation of the tissues that connect the wall of the hoof to the pedal bone in the hoof. Caused by eating too much grass, a result of infection, side effect of some drugs	Growth rings on the wall of the hoof, flared out toes, walking gingerly, higher temperature of the wall and sole.	Drugs, hoof trimming.
Equine metabolic syndrome	Caused by insulin resistance that means higher level of glucose in the blood which leads to abnormal fat deposits in the neck, shoulder, head and above the eyes.	Fat deposits as described, obesity and difficulty losing weight, excessive thirst	Balanced diet and exercise.

Some vitamins are harmful if taken in excess. Vitamins that can be harmful in excessive quantities are the fat-soluble ones: A, D, E and K.

All minerals can also be dangerous if taken in excess.

In addition to the nutritional disorders listed above, there may be some others that are specific to your chosen species. Ensure that you are familiar with them.

Activity

Research the common nutritional disorders that affect your chosen species. In each case ensure that you are familiar with their causes, signs and treatment.

Quiz Questions

1 What is the mineral calcium essential for?

2 What are a) the causes and b) the signs of vitamin D deficiency?

3 a) What is the name of a protein that cats cannot synthesise themselves? b) What are the symptoms if it is deficient?

4 What is the name of a fatty acid that cats cannot synthesise themselves? b) What are the symptoms if it is deficient?

5 What is urolithiasis and how can it be treated?

6 What are the a) causes, and b) symptoms of diabetes?

LO4 Recognise how to deliver and record basic animal treatments

4.1 How to deliver a range of basic routine and non-routine animal treatments safely, in line with codes of practice and legislation

In this topic you will learn about basic routine treatments including:

- administering medicine, sourcing treatments from qualified people and assessing for adverse reactions.

You will also learn about non-routine animal treatments, i.e. first aid, including

- the limitations and responsibilities of first aid

- classification and assessment of first aid situations, and examination of injured animals

- the identification and purpose of items in a first aid box

- the appropriate actions to take in a range of common first aid situations

- bandaging techniques, cleaning wounds, handling and restraint, and working with unpredictable animals.

Basic routine treatments

Routes of medicine administration

These include:

- Topical: these are treatments applied to the surface of the body, such as the skin or eyes. These treatments include creams, lotions, shampoos.

- Enteral: these are treatments that pass through the oesophagus, stomach or intestines. In practice this means medication given by mouth (also known as 'PO') either in feed, water, tablets etc. It can also include treatments given rectally.

- Parenteral: these are treatments that are internal but do not pass into the stomach etc. They include injections into a vein (intravenous or IV), muscle (intramuscular or IM), or under the skin (subcutaneous or SC).

Jargon Buster
topical a treatment applied to the surface of the body

enteral a treatment given internally via the mouth or rectum

parenteral a treatment given internally via injections in the skin, veins or muscles

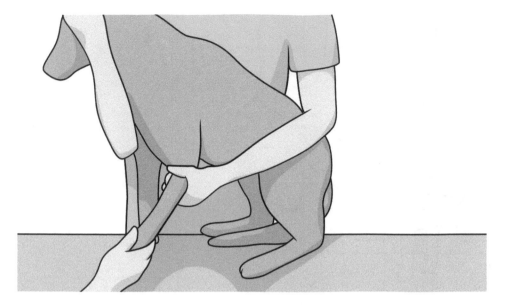

Figure 3.8 To administer an IV injection in a dog, one person restrains and presents the foreleg, whilst the second person locates the vein using their thumb

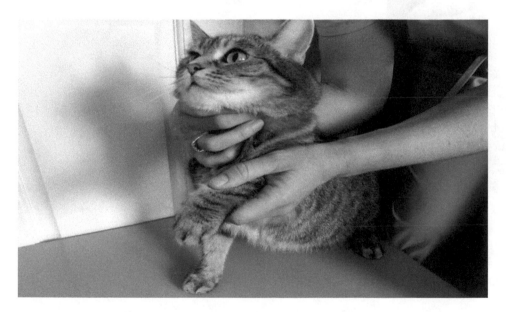

Figure 3.9 To administer an IV injection in a cat, one person restrains and presents the foreleg for a second person to lotcate the vein using their thumb

For dogs and cats

Use the foreleg for intravenous injections.

For intramuscular injections use the quadriceps muscle (at the front of the back leg) or the triceps muscle in the front leg. Do not use the hamstring (muscle at the back of the back leg).

For a subcutaneous injection locate some loose skin – this can often be found around the scruff of the neck.

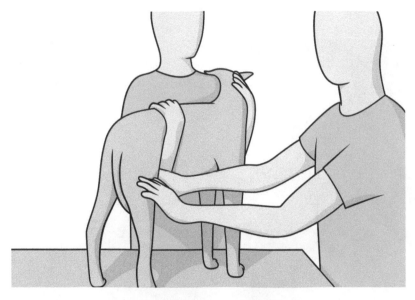

Figure 3.10 Intramuscular injection into rear leg

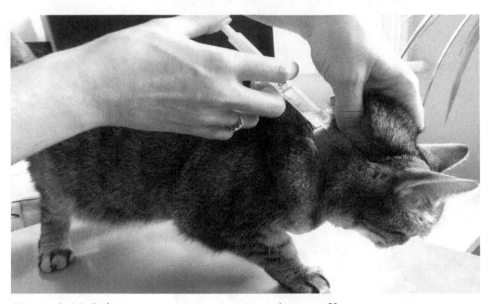

Figure 3.11 Subcutaneous injection into the scruff

Frequency of drug administration

This depends upon the choice of drug and how it is administered. Common abbreviations (from Latin, which is why they look a little strange) are:

- SID or s.i.d – once a day

- BID or b.i.d or BD – twice a day

- TID or tid – three times per day

- QID or q.i.d – four times per day

- PRN – according to need

- Qxh – once every x hours

- Qxd – once every x days

Sourcing treatments

Only certain people are legally allowed to administer certain animal medicines, know as **Registered Qualified Persons** (**RQPs**).

Vets

Veterinary medicine can only be carried out in the UK by licensed professionals, know as veterinary surgeons or vets. This is enshrined in law. Vets are licensed by the Royal College of Veterinary Surgeons.

Pharmacists

Pharmacists are professionally qualified people who are registered by the General Pharmaceutical Council or the Pharmaceutical Society of Northern Ireland. Veterinary pharmacists have permission to dispense certain medicines for animals in line with their legal responsibilities.

SQPs

Suitably Qualified Persons (**SQPs**) are entitled to prescribe or supply some animal medicinal products under the Veterinary Medicines Regulations. To qualify as an SQP requires training and examinations that lead to inclusion on an approved register. The register is kept by the Animal Medicines Training Regulatory Authority (AMTRA)

www.amtra.org.uk

There are different categories of SQP depending on which qualifications they took. This determines which types of animals they are allowed to prescribe to — farm, equine or companion.

The legal restrictions on administering animal medicines are as follows:

- POM-V prescription-only medicines can only be prescribed by a veterinary surgeon after a clinical examination.

- POM-VPS prescription-only medicines that can be prescribed by a veterinary surgeon, pharmacist or SQP.

- NFA-VPS (Non-food animal): does not require a prescription but can only be supplied by a veterinary surgeon, pharmacist or SQP.

- AVM-GSL Authorised veterinary medicine – general sales list: there are no legal restrictions to suplying these medicines.

Small animal exception scheme: certain small animals, if kept as pets, are exempt from some of the restrictions above; but some medicines are still restricted – particularly antibiotics, narcotics and psychotropics.

Feed merchants

Some medicine can be administered via animal feed – however such administration must be in line with the legal requirements above, regarding RQPs

> **Jargon Buster**
> narcotic a drug that dulls the senses and induces sleep
>
> psychotropic a drug that affects mental state

Assessing animals for adverse reactions

An adverse reaction is one which is harmful and unintended when medication is used at the correct dose. Adverse reactions to medication is very rare as the UK market is strictly regulated. It is therefore important to know what to do and who to tell if there is a reaction.

You should report the issue to the Veterinary Medicines Directorate. They have an online reporting system where you can describe the issue. Alternatively you can report the issued to the marketing authorisation holder (MAH), or distributor of the products, who are legally obliged to report the issue to the VMD.

Anaphylaxis is a rare but serious allergic reaction that may sometimes be in response to medicine. Symptoms include itchy, red or swollen skin, sudden onset of vomiting or diarrhoea, and difficulties in breathing. The condition should be treated as an emergency: blood pressure will need to be monitored and maintained, airways to remain clear and adrenalin may need to be injected intravenously.

Animals should always be monitored after any treatment, adverse reactions assessed for severity and treated appropriately.

Non-routine animal treatments

Aims, rules and limitations of first aid

First aid is the immediate help and care given to an acutely ill or injured animal. The aims of first aid are to:

- preserve life
- protect from further harm
- reduce pain and suffering
- promote recovery.

In extreme cases, providing the correct care quickly can mean the difference between life and death, or a full and partial recovery. However first aid is limited to ensuring the best possible outcome for the animal before full medical help from a veterinary surgeon can be given. It does not involve diagnosing what might be the cause of the illness.

It must be remembered that it is illegal for anyone other than a vet to perform medical procedures on an animal. Therefore first aid that is performed by anyone else is strictly limited to the aims outlined above.

Classification of first aid situations

Minor

These are conditions where first aid can either deal with the problem entirely or keep the animal comfortable until a suitable appointment with a vet. e.g.:

- superficial wounds i.e. scratches and cuts that are not deep

Jargon Buster

pharmacovigilance monitoring and evaluation of adverse reactions to medicine

anaphylaxis a severe allergic reaction that can lead to life-threatening breathing difficulties

(however if the injuries were from a fight with another animal then antibiotics may need to be given.)

- mild heatstroke
- minor allergies
- insect bites or stings.

Immediate

These are conditions that are not life-threatening but require prompt attention to either stabilise the situation or make the animal comfortable. A vet will need to be seen promptly, e.g.:

- any non-superficial wounds
- bone fractures, dislocations and breaks
- any wounds or problems with the eyes.

Life-threatening

These are conditions in which the animal is likely to die unless immediate intervention is made and a vet will need to be seen immediately e.g.:

- poisoning
- severe burns
- severe wounds
- uncontrolled bleeding
- severe allergic reaction
- obstructions to the airway
- severe breathing problems
- weak pulse
- animal is unconscious.

Assessing the first aid situation and examination of an injured animal

If you are confronted with a first aid situation, you need to assess if it is a minor, immediate or life-threatening situation. Life-threatening situations clearly need immediate action. However, in all cases you should:

- Stay calm.
- Get help as soon as possible by contacting a vet.
- Ensure you are not putting yourself or others at further risk before taking any action.
- Check that airways are clear, that the animal is breathing, and that their circulation (pulse) is normal.
- Stop any bleeding.

- You may need to treat the animal for shock.

Be aware that animals in pain or distress may be aggressive towards you, which may cause you an injury and further harm them. This is the case even for animals that are normally very friendly and docile. You will need to consider restraining and/or muzzling before handling.

When assessing or examining an animal you will need to stay very calm - remember the animal is likely to be frightened. You can try to soothe them as much as possible by talking quietly and reassuringly, and being careful to make no sudden movements. You should try not to touch or move the animal unless it is strictly necessary.

First Aid box contents

- **Selection of bandages**

- **Adhesive tape**

Used to dress wounds and keep them clean.

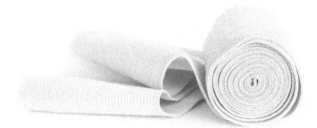

- **Cotton wool**

- **Sterile dressing materials**

Cotton wool can be used for padding and dressing material is used on the site of a wound.

Figure 3.12 Bandages and adhesive tape

- **Rectal thermometer (plus lubricant)**

For accurate temperature measurement – see LO1.

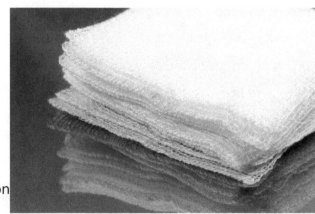

- **Tweezers**

to remove thorns, splinters, stings

- **Gloves, hand sanitizer**

to prevent cross-contamination and for protection against infections and chemicals used in treatments/medicines

Figure 3.13 Cotton wool and dressing material

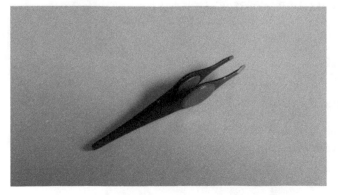

Figure 3.14 Tweezers

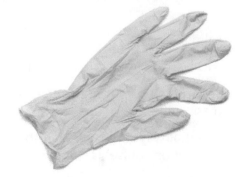

Figure 3.15 Gloves and hand sanitisers

• **Scissors**

for cutting bandages, tape, dressing material or fur

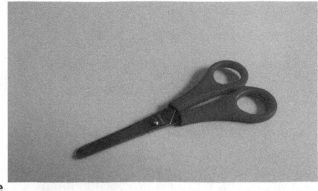

Figure 3.16 Scissors

• **Eye wash, antiseptic solution**

in case of debris in the eye

• **Contact details for the local veterinary practice**

vital in an emergency

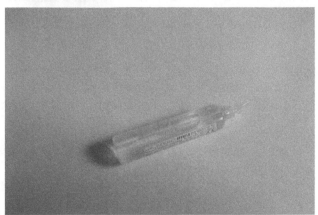

Figure 3.17 Eye-wash

• **Carrier bag**

• **Blanket**

to help keep animals warm after an incident but can also be used as a makeshift stretcher

• **Poultice**

A soft moist compound that is applied to the skin to draw out infections. These are commercially available.

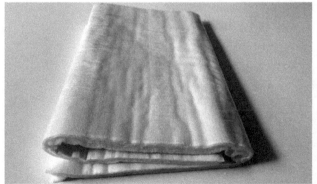

Figure 3.18 A poultice

Figure 3.19 Blanket

Common first aid situations and appropriate actions

Shock

Shock is a lack of blood supply to the major organs and/or brain. It can be triggered by a range of events but it is more than simply 'being shocked'. It is a life-threatening condition and needs to be treated immediately. Symptoms include white gums, faint quick heartbeat, quick breaths, being cold to the touch, and a slow capillary refill time.

There are different stages and severities of shock and the aim with first aid is to prevent the condition escalating to the next more serious stage. Treatment normally includes:

- keeping the animal warm

- preventing any blood loss

- keeping airways clear

- stopping the animal from moving around

- keeping the head lower than the body.

Road Traffic Collision (RTC)

Before attempting to help an injured animal you must make sure that the situation is safe for you and other road users. You need to make sure that the road is free of traffic or that other cars have sufficient warning of an incident to ensure they are not putting you in danger.

The sooner a vet can help the better, so ensure you or someone else phones a vet's emergency number as soon as possible.

- Be careful when approaching the animal as it may bite if injured or distressed. If the animal is not having difficulty breathing then it might be safer to use a temporary muzzle, constructed from bandages in your first aid kit.

- Be calm, gentle and soothing with the animal – you don't want to cause it further distress.

- Check the A-B-C:

  * Airway – ensure the airway is not blocked and lie the animal in the recovery position.

  * Breathing – if breathing has stopped be prepared to administer respiratory assistance – either chest compressions or mouth-to-nose resuscitation.

  * Circulation – check the pulse and be prepared to administer chest compressions to get the heart beating again.

- If the animal is bleeding try and stop the flow of blood by compressing the wound.

- Cover any wounds.

- The parcel shelf from a car can be used for a stretcher for animals with suspected broken bones – particularly the spine. Alternatively a blanket can be used.

- Get the animal to the vet as soon as possible.

Convulsions

Also known as 'fits' or 'seizures', these result from abnormal electrical activity in the brain which interferes with the normal processes. There can be many different reasons for the abnormal activity but it will result in a lack of control of the muscles. This might mean the animal goes quite still and can't seem to move, or might lead to wild and uncontrolled movements.

- The main danger to the animal is that they hurt themselves whilst they are having a convulsion. So move any object out of the way that may provide a danger. If possible wrap the animal in a blanket.

- Keep noise to a minimum.

- Try not to touch the animal.

- Do not put anything near the animal's mouth and do not attempt to give them food or water.

- If the seizure lasts for more than a few minutes then call a vet.

Fractures

A fracture is a name for a broken bone. However the break might be a full break or an incomplete one. A fracture can be relatively simple if there is a complete break and there is no damage to the surrounding area. However more complicated fractures are when the broken bone penetrates the skin (i.e. you can see the bone), or causes internal bleeding.

A bone may be fractured if the animal is having trouble walking, can't put weight on a leg, is unwilling to allow you to touch a part of their body, or has limbs that are positioned in an unnatural way.

If the animal has a fracture it is probably in pain and may bite – so ensure it is restrained and muzzled if necessary.

- Keep the animal calm.

- If the fracture has broken the skin then there may be bleeding, in which case try to stop it and cover any open wounds with a sterile dressing.

- Try to stop the animal from moving the affected bone(s). For the legs and tail this can be achieved by applying a splint. For other bones you should try and stop the animal from moving.

- Do not try and reposition any bones – you may cause further damage.

- Take them to a vet as soon as possible.

Wounds

If there is an open wound (i.e. the skin is broken) and is still bleeding, cover with a dressing material and apply pressure until the bleeding stops. Do not remove the dressing once the bleeding has stopped. Ensure that there are no objects in the wound before applying pressure.

If the open wound is minor and not bleeding, clean the wound using an antiseptic and then dress and cover.

Closed wounds are when the skin has not been broken but there is damage to the tissue underneath. Treatment aims to prevent further tissue damage. This can be done using a cold compress, by applying ice wrapped in a towel to the affected area.

Dislocations

This is when a bone has been taken out of position at the joint. The animal may find it painful to move the joint, and the joint and bone may just look 'wrong'. It can be difficult to see the difference between a fracture and a dislocation.

- To stop the animal moving the affected bones follow the same guidelines as for fractures.
- Putting a bone back into the correct position should be left to a vet.

Choking

An animal can only survive for a matter of minutes if unable to breathe, so immediate action needs to be taken for animals that are choking.

- Restrain the animal and check the airway for any obvious blockages (including the tongue).
- If the blockage does not come out then you can grasp both hands just below the rib cage and pull them sharply towards you. This has the affect of expelling breath, which can dislodge the object. You must be very careful, particularly with smaller animals, as the wrong hand position can break bones.

Poisoning

Animals can be poisoned through eating or breathing in a toxic substance, or through exposure to the skin. If you think an animal has been poisoned then the first thing is to establish what the poison is. Remember that poison means any substance that is toxic for an animal – this can include everyday items such as chocolate, raisins and houseplants.

Some symptoms of poisoning are:

- stomach pain
- unsteady on the feet
- salivating, vomiting
- slow capillary refill time.

If an animal has been exposed or eaten something poisonous then take action immediately – don't wait for symptoms to appear.

- Do not induce vomiting.
- Keep the animal warm and comfortable.
- Place in the recovery position.
- Note down the likely source of the poison if known.
- Get them to a vet immediately.

Burns and scalds

Burns can range from first degree (mild) to third degree (severe). A vet will need to be consulted for second and third degree burns. But for all burns you should:

- restrain the animal
- cool the area by applying a cloth soaked in cold water

- do not apply any creams or ointments
- do not break any blisters
- see a vet immediately for second and third degree burns.

Bites and stings

Bites normally result in open wounds where there is a risk of infection. Refer to the guidelines for open wounds.

Stings from insects can be painful and result in red, itchy and swollen skin.

- If the sting is still in the animal then try and remove it, taking care not to break it.
- Apply ice or a cold compress to the sting, for pain relief.

Foreign bodies

If items have penetrated the skin then:

- do not remove the item
- reduce the size of the item so that it protrudes by only a few centimetres
- restrict the movement of the animal
- attempt to control any bleeding but do not push the object further into the skin
- see a vet immediately.

If any foreign objects have embedded themselves in the eye then do not try and remove them. Prevent the animal from touching its own eye and see a vet immediately.

Haemorrhages

Haemorrhages – heavy bleeding – is dangerous because an animal can lose a lot of blood quickly. This can lead to shock, or it can lead to tissue damage. If it is external then heavy bleeding is obvious; but there might be internal bleeding which is not obvious. Symptoms of non-visible bleeding are:

- pale gums
- rapid pulse and/or breath
- slow capillary refill time
- coughing up blood, or blood present in the faeces.

For external bleeding the main aim is to reduce or stop the bleeding:

- place a clean absorbent dressing material onto the affected point
- make sure there are no foreign objects in the wound
- press on the dressing with your fingers for up to 10 minutes.

Alternatively, or additionally, you could apply a tourniquet or pressure bandage to a limb or tail to constrict the flow of blood to the affected area. The tourniquet can be left in place for 15 minutes.

Another alternative is to locate the nearest artery that supplies the affected area and apply pressure there to slow or stop blood flowing to the affected area.

Restricting blood flow in any of these ways is only a temporary measure because a lack of blood to the tissues will cause long-term problems - so you should consult a vet immediately in all cases of heavy bleeding.

Common techniques

You will need to demonstrate the following:

- bandaging techniques
- cleaning wounds
- precautions for working with an unpredictable animal
- handling and restraint techniques.

Bandaging techniques

Bandaging normally consists of several different layers:

Dressing layer: if there is a wound then the first layer is to dress the wound. As it is in direct contact with the skin this layer should not be adhesive, as it will stick and cause further damage to the skin (and pain) when removing.

Primary or padding layer: this layer provides protection and padding to the area.

Secondary layer: normally a layer adapts to the shape of the body (conforms) so it can hold the whole thing in place.

Tertiary layer: for further support and to provide a final layer of protection.

To bandage a paw (figure 3.20):

- A Add a primary layer of padding between the toes and around the animal's pads.

- B Starting above the front of the foot, roll further padding over and under the foot to the back of the ankle, and then back again to the starting position so that there are two layers of bandage.

- C Then diagonally overlap and roll the padding down the leg to the bottom of the foot and back again.

- D Add the final tertiary layer by wrapping the foot as per instruction B.

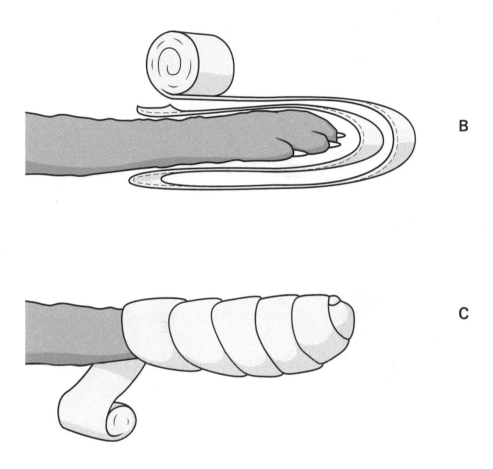

B

C

Figure 3.20 Bandaging a paw

Bandaging limbs (figure 3.21):

The Robert Jones bandage method is often used for limbs and is as follows:

- A Add padding between the toes and pads.

- B Attach two strips of zinc oxide tape to the front and back of the leg, leaving an overhang of around 10cm.

- C Wrap a strip of cotton wool in spirals around the leg, starting from the foot. Leave a gap for the claws to poke out. Wrap the cotton wool at least four times around the leg, so that it is much wider than normal.

- D Apply a conformal bandage as the second layer over the cotton wool.

- E Attach the zinc oxide tapes to the second layer and then wrap in conforming tape as the tertiary layer.

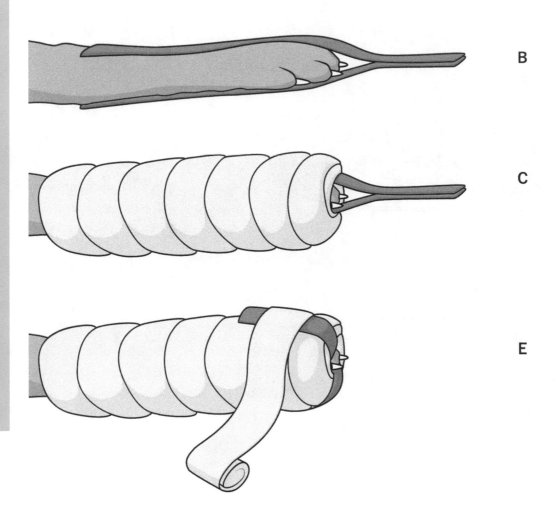

B

C

E

Figure 3.21 Bandaging limbs

Bandaging ear/head (figure 3.22):

- A If there is a wound on the ear then dress it.

- B Fold the ear back onto the head and hold in the most comfortable and natural position.

- C Starting at the injured ear, wrap a cohesive bandage around the head twice: under the chin, behind the other ear, across the injured ear, back under the chin, and then in front of the other ear, until you reach the injured ear again.

- D Then wrap a padding layer around the head and ear, following the same pattern as for the bandage i.e. under the chin and in front/ behind the other ear.

- E Apply a conforming bandage, again following the same pattern as before.

- F Add the top layer self-adhesive bandage and tape the ends.

- G Ensure that the uninjured ear is free and that bandage is not covering the eyes.

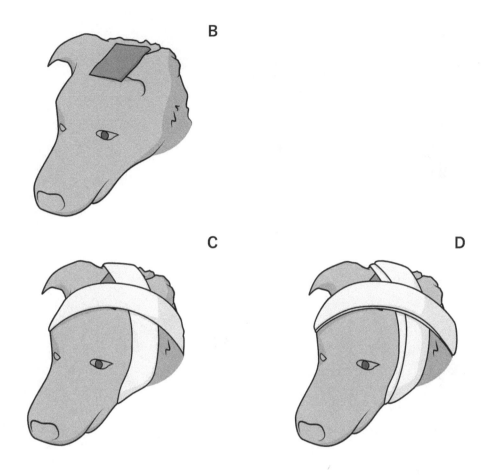

Figure 3.22 Bandaging ear/head

Bandaging abdomen (figure 3.23):

- A A colleague may need to restrain the standing animal whilst you apply the bandages.

- B If there are any wounds then dress them.

- C Wrap a bandage around the chest and abdomen, going under the ribs and stomach and across the back, ensuring that the bandage overlaps each time it goes around. Continue wrapping until the entire chest and abdomen is covered.

- D Using the same bandage, wrap between the front legs and then pass over one shoulder, and then repeat.

- E Now repeat but for the other shoulder, and then stick the bandage with tape.

- F You can apply some padding if needed.

- G Then wrap a cohesive outer layer, following the same wrapping pattern as before. Attach the end of the bandage with tape.

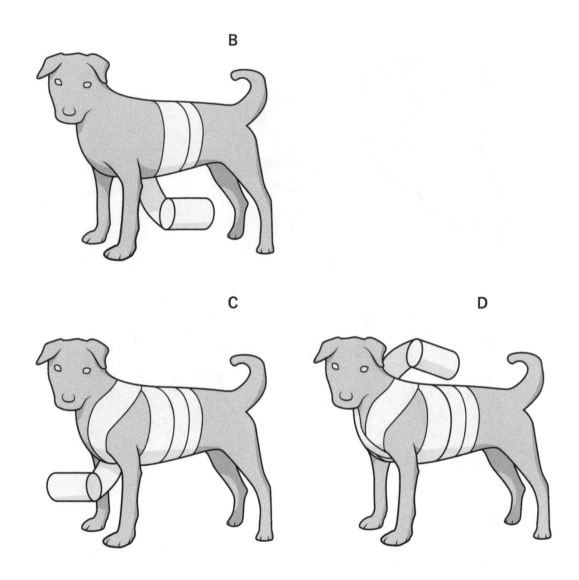

Figure 3.23 Bandaging an abdomen

Bandaging a tail (figure 3.24):

- A Apply any dressing and consider taping to keep it place.

- B Apply a padding layer by covering the length of the tail, over the tip and then back under the length of the tail. Then wrap the padding around the circumference of the tail, covering the padding you had already applied and overlapping by about 1/3, going to the tip of the tail and back to the body. Repeat by going down and up the tail again.

- C Following the same pattern as above, apply the conformal bandage.

- D Add a top layer following the same pattern.

B

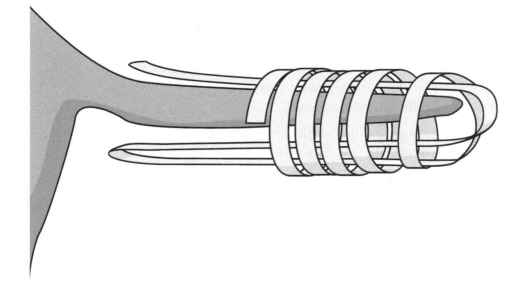

Figure 3.24 Bandaging a tail

Cleaning of wounds

An open wound is when the skin has been broken – a cut, graze, abrasion etc. Only an open wound needs cleaning.

- Before cleaning ensure the wound has stopped bleeding.

- All non-surgical wounds will contain bacteria which need to be destroyed to encourage speedy healing and prevent further problems.

- Use a saline solution, made from a teaspoon of salt in a pint of lukewarm water, to generously wash the wound to disinfect and remove debris. If there is still some visible dirt, grit or other substances in the wound, use a soft cloth bathed in the saline solution to gently clean the wound.

- Dry the wound and dress it.

Instead of a saline solution you can use an antibacterial solution recommended for the animal you are working with. Note that some antibacterial products for humans are not suitable for animals.

Consideration of working with an unpredictable animal and precautions to take

Any animal in pain may behave unpredictably, even one that is normally completely placid. It is therefore important to consider your own safety before approaching an animal that you suspect is ill or has sustained any kind of injury.

- Avoid surprising an animal. Do not approach from a blind-spot or behind it and move slowly and predictably. Do not corner the animal.

- Ensure your full attention is on the animal at all times but avoid direct eye contact.

- Be aware of behavioural signs that show the animal is stressed, angry or aggressive. These will differ between species.

- Crouch down so you are on their level but do not sit down. Ensure that you are free to move away easily and quickly if required.

- Wear protective equipment if necessary.

- Use a calm and gentle tone.

- Ensure the animal is handled and restrained correctly – see below.

The use of handling and restraint techniques and equipment

None-contact: Some trained animals may respond to verbal commands or physical gestures.

Mice and rats: May be held up by the base of the tail – but not for an extended period of time. You can also hold the base of the tail with one hand and grasp the back of the neck with the other.

Rabbits: Grasp the scruff of the neck and gently lift whilst using your other arm to cradle and support the back and hind legs. Never pick a rabbit up by its ears.

Cats: You can use one hand to restrain the head with the other restraining the body. Alternatively you can grasp the scruff of the neck with one hand to restrain. If these techniques do not work then you can place a heavy towel over the cat to restrain it, taking care to ensure all limbs are inside the towel.

Dogs: Collars and leads are the most common restraint method used for dogs and indeed most dogs will be familiar with wearing them.

Muzzles will stop a dog from biting. You can create a muzzle by looping a suitably strong cloth or bandage in the same way as you tie a shoelace (before you create the bow). Place the dog's snout inside the loop and then pull both ends to tighten (figure 3.25). Bring the ends under the chin and then round the back of the dog's neck and tie off into a bow. Do not leave a muzzle on for an extended period of time.

For very aggressive dogs you may need to consider a restraint pole, which ensures the animal is kept at a safe distance.

If there is no risk of being bitten, you can lift a dog in different ways, depending on its size:

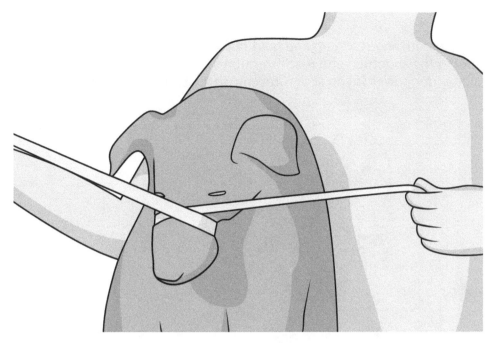

Figure 3.25 Muzzling a dog

small dog – place one arm under the dog's head and the other hand under the abdomen with your fingers between the front legs (figure 3.26).

large dog – requires two people to lift, the first restraining the dog's head with one arm and the other behind the top of the front legs; the second person places one arm underneath the abdomen and the other arm under the tail around the back legs (figure 3.27).

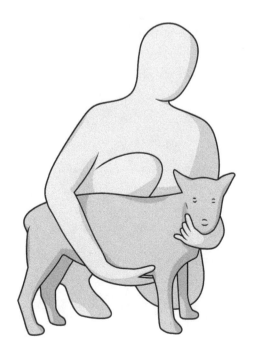

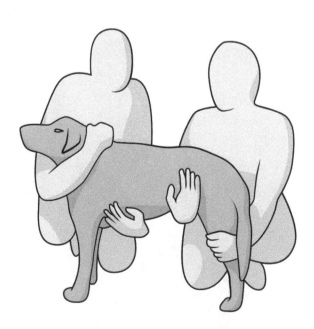

Figure 3.26 Lifting a small dog   *Figure 3.27 Lifting a large dog*

Restraining whilst standing up

Place one arm underneath the mouth and reach up and hold the neck; place the other arm underneath the abdomen and reach through to hold the back and then pull the dog towards you so it is resting against your body (figure 3.28).

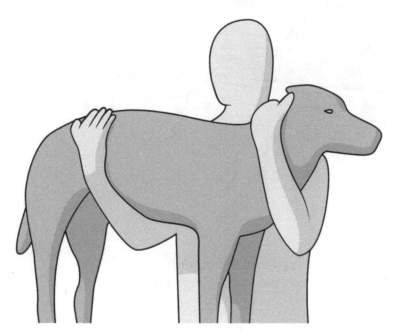

Figure 3.28 Restraining a standing dog

Restraining whilst sitting down

Place one hand over the back and rear haunches to ensure the dog sits down, and the place the other arm underneath the mouth and reach up to hold the neck. Pull the dog towards you so it is resting against your body (figure 3.29).

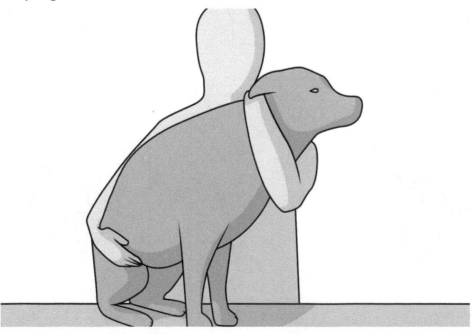

Figure 3.29 Restraining a sitting dog

Restraining whilst laying down

Lay the dog down on its side on a table, so that its back is resting against your body, then reach over and grasp both front paws, using your arm to push lightly on the base of the dog's neck. Reach over with your other arm and grasp both rear paws (figure 3.30).

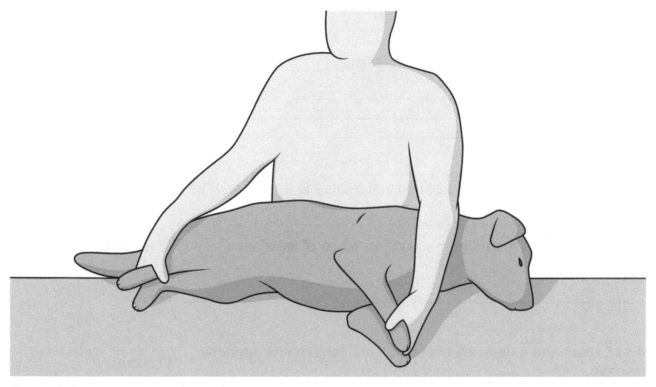

Figure 3.30 Restraining a lying dog

Quiz Questions

1 What could you use to restrain an aggressive dog?

2 Outline how you would treat an open wound.

3 What is the first thing you should do if an animal has been involved in a road traffic collision?

4 What are two signs of an internal haemorrhage?

5 Explain how you would treat shock.

6 Name three items you would expect to find in a first aid box.

7 What are the aims of first aid?

8 Name two life-threatening first aid conditions.

END OF UNIT QUESTIONS

1 State **two** health checks that you would carry out every day.

(1) mark

_____

2 List **three** different pathogenic organisms.

(3 marks)

_____
_____
_____

3 a) Name **one** piece of legislation that relates to animal health.   (1 mark)

_____

b) Describe the aim and purpose of this piece of legislation.   (2 marks)

_____
_____

4 a) Explain the difference between a notifiable and a zoonotic disease.

(1 mark)

_____

b) State **two** notifiable diseases.

(2 marks)

_____
_____

c) Describe the actions that should be taken if an animal is suspected of having a zoonotic disease.   (4 marks)

_____
_____
_____
_____

5 a) State a disease that a rabbit should be vaccinated against.

(1 mark)

_____

b) When and how often should this vaccine be given?

(2 marks)

_____
_____

6 a) State a disease that is spread through direct transmission. (1 mark)

_____

b) Describe the implications of a directly transmitted disease? (4 marks)

_____
_____
_____

7 a) State **one** common vitamin deficiency and **one** common mineral deficiency. (2 marks)

_____
_____

b) For each one, describe the causes and symptoms of the deficiency. (4 marks)

_____
_____
_____

8 Describe the difference between a pharmacist and a suitably qualified person. (2 marks)

_____
_____

9 Describe the actions that should and should not be taken if a cat is suspected of having been poisoned. (6 marks)

_____
_____
_____
_____
_____
_____
_____
_____

10 List **three** considerations that should be taken when working with an unpredictable animal. (3 marks)

_____
_____
_____
_____

Unit 304 Animal Feeding and Nutrition

LO1 Understand the basics of nutrition

1.1 Contribution of the major nutrients of an animal's diet to maintain health and wellbeing

In this topic you will learn about the major nutrients required for a balanced diet:

- carbohdyrates
- proteins
- fats/lipids
- vitamins
- minerals
- water.

Carbohydrates

Carbohydrates are molecules made up of carbon, hydrogen and oxygen atoms. They are an important source of energy for animals. There are three main types of carbohydrates: monosaccharides, disaccharides and polysaccharides.

Monosaccharides

These have the simplest chemical structures and are often called simple sugars. They include glucose, galactose and fructose. All three of these are absorbed quickly and easily by the body after eating. Glucose is the main energy source for the body, and most carbohydrates are broken down into glucose during the digestion process, which has the effect of raising blood sugar levels. Monosaccharides are found naturally in fruit and honey, and they are added to all sorts of foodstuff to sweeten them.

Disaccharides

Two monosaccharides can combine to create a disaccharide. Examples are sucrose (common sugar), lactose and maltose. Disaccharides are known as sugars (but note they are not 'simple').

Sucrose is made from the monosaccharides glucose and fructose.

Lactose is made from the monosaccharides glucose and galactose and is found in milk.

Maltose is made up of two monosaccharide glucose molecules.

Polysaccharides

Many monosaccharides joined together are called polysaccharides – and are also known as complex carbohydrates. Common polysaccharides include starch, glycogen and cellulose.

Starch is found in lots of foodstuff, such as rice, cereals, grains and bread. Starch is made from a form of glucose called alpha-glucose. It is broken down into glucose during digestion but because it is a complex carbohydrate, the process takes much longer than for mono- or disaccharides.

Glycogen is created in the body from glucose and is essentially a store of energy. When the body needs energy it can draw upon its glycogen stores and break it down into glucose.

Cellulose is made from beta-glucose. It makes up the cell walls in plants. It is a structure that gives vegetables their 'crunch' but it cannot be digested by humans or most animals. However ruminants – cloven-hoofed animals such as cows, sheep, goats, deer – have a chamber in their stomach containing bacteria and protozoa that can break down cellulose into fatty acids which is then digestible. (For more on this see page 76.) Through this mechanism cellulose is the main source of energy for ruminants. For all other animals cellulose is still useful because it acts a source of dietary fibre – something which aids the digestion process.

(For more on this see page 76.)

> **Jargon Buster**
> **monsaccharide** the simplest carbohydrates, e.g. glucose and fructose
>
> **disaccharide** two monosaccharides joined together e.g. sucrose
>
> **polysaccharide** many monosaccharides joined together, also known as complex carbohydrates e.g.starch and cellulose

a) i) alpha-glucose   a) ii) beta-glucose   b) maltose

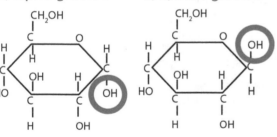

c) starch - made from alpha-glucose molecules

d) cellulose - made from beta-glucose molecules

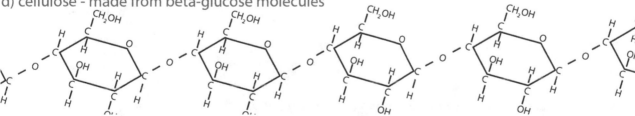

Figure 4.1 a) Glucose is a monosaccharide that comes in two forms - alpha and beta. The difference between them is circled in red. b) Maltose is a disacharride made from two glucose molecules. c) Starch is a polysaccharide made from many alpha-glucose molecules. d) Cellulose is a polysaccharide made from many beta-glucose molecules.

65

Proteins

Amino acids are small molecules that are essential for life. Peptide is a catch-all term for the combination of two or more amino acids. A dipeptide is specific term for when two amino acids combine. If three or more amino acids combine then they are known as polypetides. Very long chains of 50 or more amino acids are called proteins.

In nutrition, however, the word 'protein' is often used as a catch-all term to refer to peptides, polypeptides and actual proteins. So we will do the same here too.

There are 21 different amino acids which can make up proteins that human and animals need. Different proteins have a different sequence of amino acids. Proteins are workhorses of the body and perform many different functions at a cellular level.

Animal (and human) bodies can make (or synthesise) many amino acids but not all of them. The amino acids that cannot be synthesised must be obtained through food instead, and are known as essential amino acids. Different species may have different requirements – for instance cats are unable to synthesise one amino acid that other species can, and therefore what is essential in the diet for a cat is not essential for, say, a dog. The dietary requirements of a cat are therefore different to those of a dog.

Essential amino acids can be obtained from both plant and animal sources – fish, meat, dairy, pulses and cereals.

Proteins can also be used by the body as a source of energy if other sources – e.g. carbohydrates and fat – have run out. Excess protein is not stored in the body, however, and is instead converted into urea and excreted from the body in urine.

Jargon Buster

amino acid organic molecules that are essential for life

peptide a combination of amino acides

dipeptide a combination of two amino acids

polypeptide a combination of ten or more amino acids

protein a combination of 50 or more amino acids, proteins are involved in almost all structures and functions of the body

essential amino acids amino acids that a species is unable to make themselves and thus must be obtained through food sources

a) All amino acids are made up of hydrogen, carbon, nitrogen and oxygen. R is different for each amino acid and represents different molecules in each case.

b) The simplest amino acid is glycine; R in this case is hydrogen. Bonding two glycine molecules together forms the dipeptide glycylglycine (and water is given off as a by product).

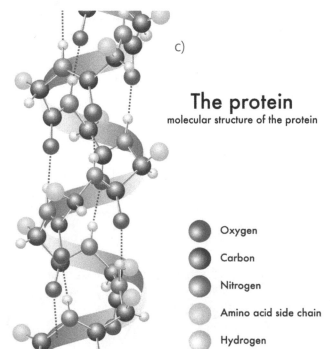

c)

The protein
molecular structure of the protein

● Oxygen

● Carbon

● Nitrogen

○ Amino acid side chain

○ Hydrogen

Figure 4.2 Chemical structure of a) amino acid, b) dipeptide, c) protein

Fats and lipids

A group of molecules known as fatty acids consist of long chains of hydrogen and carbon atoms, arranged in different ways. Fatty acids chemically combine with a molecule called glycerol to form fats. Because there are many different types of fatty acid that can combine with glycerol, there are many different types of fat.

In nutrition lipid is sometimes used as an interchangeable term with fat. However in biochemistry lipid is a broader term that includes fatty acids, as well as fat. So fat is really a subset of a broader set of substances called lipids.

Fats are classified as **saturated** or **unsaturated**, according to the chemical bonding structure of the fatty acids that they are made from. Unsaturated fatty acids have at least one double bond between carbon atoms whereas saturated fats do not have any double bonds. Saturated fats are solid at room temperature and usually found in meat and dairy products. Unsaturated fats are liquid at room temperature and are usually found in vegetable products and fish. Saturated animal fats are created from unsaturated fats in plant material, in a process called hydrogenation, by bacteria within an animal's gut.

Fats are a concentrated form of energy and can be stored under the skin. Fats are also essential to the absorption of vitamins A, D, E and K. The body needs certain fatty acids, known as essential fatty acids. Examples include linolenic acid, linoleic acid and arachidonic acid. Dogs can synthesise arachidonic acid from other fatty acids; cats however cannot and must obtain it from their diet. Arachidonic acid is only found in animal fats.

Fats provide insulation for animals and protects their internal organs from external impact. Animals adapted to living in deserts - e.g. kangaroo rats - also use fat stores to create water (known as metabolic water). Certain types of fats are also important elements within cell membranes.

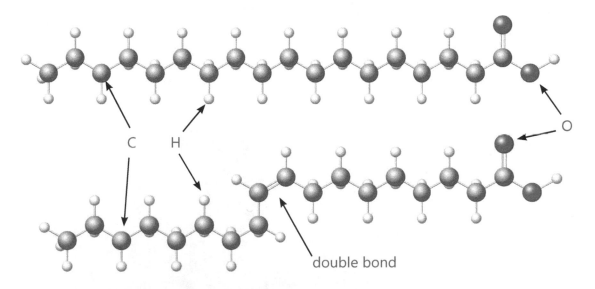

C   H

double bond

Figure 4.3 Chemical structure of fatty acids: a) (Top) saturated animal fat (stearic acid) b) (Bottom) unsaturated vegetable fat (oleic acid, from olive oil) - note the double bond.

Vitamins and minerals

For a full list of vitamins and minerals see Unit 303 Section 2.4.

Water

Water does not provide any nutrition for animals. However water is essential for animal life because it:

- provides a medium in which chemical reactions can take place
- delivers nutrients to the body's cells
- is used to flush toxins away from the body
- regulates body temperature.

Continuous availability of fresh water is critical to the health of animals.

Quiz Questions

1 a) What are the three main types of carbohydrate, and b) what role do carbohydrates play in nutrition?

2 a) What are proteins made up of, and b) what role do proteins play in nutrition?

3 Name two things that fat is important for.

4 Name two functions that water provides.

1.2 Functions of the major nutrients within the animal's body

In this topic you will learn about the functions of the major nutrients, to include:

• energy

• growth and repair

• storage and insulation

	Carbohydrate	Protein	Fat	Vitamins and mineral
Energy	The 'go to' source of energy. Most carbohydrates are broken down through digestive processes into glucose, which is then absorbed into the bloodstream. Cellulose, however, is only digested by ruminants and hindgut fermenters – see page 75-6. 3.5 calories per gram.	If carbohydrates and fat are not available then the body can obtain energy from protein. However this is a last resort. 3.5 calories per gram.	The body can call upon its fat reserves as an alternative source of energy. However it takes longer than carbohydrate to process. 8.5 calories per gram.	These are not sources of energy but their presence can help release energy from the other sources.
Growth and repair	Not directly involved with growth and repair. However a diet deficient in carbohydrates will source protein as a fuel and thus inhibit growth and repair indirectly.	Crucial for growth of young animals and for the on-going repair to cells necessary in adults.	No role in growth and repair.	Various vitamins and minerals play important roles in the growth and repair of bodies. See Unit 303 Section 2.4 for a detailed list.

Storage and insulation	Stored in the form of glycogen, in the liver and muscles.	Protein cannot be stored in the body.	Fat is stored in cells under the skin and around muscles. They act as a shock absorber for organs and also provide insulation.	Fat soluble vitamins (A, D, E, K) are stored in the liver. This means that too much of these vitamins in the diet can cause liver damage. B12 is water soluble but is also stored in the liver. Water soluble vitamins (rest of the B-range, C and folic acid) are not stored in the body, so dietary sources need to be regular. The body gets rid of any excess. Minerals are stored within the structure of the body itself – for instance, the skeleton contains most of the calcium in the body. However the liver is also a storage site for some minerals, e.g. iron and copper.
Consequences of consuming too much	As an energy source, the body will convert and store unused carbohydrates as fat. This can lead to putting on weight and obesity which can lead to a range of health problems.	Can lead to problems with the kidney.	The body will store unused fat, which can lead to putting on weight and obesity which can lead to a range of health problems.	Water-soluble vitamins are excreted from the body. Fat-soluble vitamins are stored in the body and overdosing on those can lead to liver problems. As the body will store mineral in its structure as well as the liver, excessive consumption of any mineral will lead to health problems. For more information on vitamins and minerals see Unit 303 Section 2.4.

Activity

Choose one fat-soluble vitamin and one mineral. Research the health consequences of consuming too much of each.

1 Which nutrient is responsible for growth and repair?

2 Where are carbohydrates stored in the body?

3 Which vitamins are stored in the liver?

4 Which nutrient contains the most amount of energy

5 Where are minerals stored in the body? Give an example.

1.3 Digestion and absorption of the major nutrients within the animal's body

In this topic you will learn about biological digestion and absorption for monogastric animals and ruminants, including:

- **biological digestion**

- **animals with monogastric stomachs, including hindgut fermenters**

- **ruminants.**

Biological digestion

The intestines consist of long coiled tubes that run from the stomach to the anus. There are three parts to the intestine: the small intestine, which absorbs nutrients from food; the large intestine, which absorbs water from the food; and the rectum, where the stools form that need to be excreted.

The tubes of the intestines are made up of the following layers (figure 4.4):

Mucosa

This is the innermost layer of the intestinal wall. It consists of:

- mucosal ducts and glands: these are located on the innermost part of the intestines, and their role is to generate mucous that covers the internal surface of the intestines.

- villi: The inner surface of the intestine is made up of tiny finger-like projections called villi, which increase the surface area in contact with the contents of the intestine. The villi contain many minute blood capillaries. Nutrients are absorbed through the villi into these blood vessels, and from there enter the blood stream.

- lacteals: The villi also contain lymphatic capillaries, known as lacteals, whose job is to absorb fat and fat-soluble vitamins, and eventually

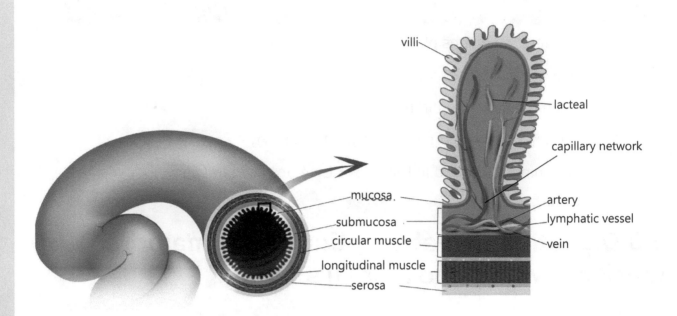

Figure 4.4 Structure of the intestines

transport these into the bloodstream. The lymph system is also there to fight infection from microorganisms. The intestines provide an entry point into the body for invaders, so this role is important.

The mechanisms for the absorption of nutrients are osmosis (across a semi-permeable membrane), diffusion (from high concentration to low concentration) and active transport (from low concentration to high concentration, requiring cellular work to achieve this).

Muscle layers

There are two different layers of muscle surrounding the mucosa. The first is a circular layer of muscle, that forms a ring around the intestine. The second layer is muscle arranged longitudinally, along the length of the intestine. The contractions of these muscles cause food to move through the intestine.

Serosa

The serosa is a smooth membrane that surrounds the intestines. It secretes a substance called serous that helps reduce friction from the muscle movement.

Monogastric stomach

Monogastric means a stomach that has only one chamber. A whole range of animals fall into this category, including humans. (This is in contrast to animals that have a four-chambered stomach, known as ruminants – for details see the next section.)

Digestive system organs

The key organs of the monogastric digestive system are:

- the tongue
- the salivary glands
- the gastrointestinal tract consisting of:
    * the mouth
    * the oesophagus
    * the stomach
    * the small intestine
    * the large intestine (also known as the colon)
- the pancreas
- the liver
- the gallbladder

> **Jargon Buster**
>
> monogastric one stomach
>
> ruminant animal with a four-chambered stomach

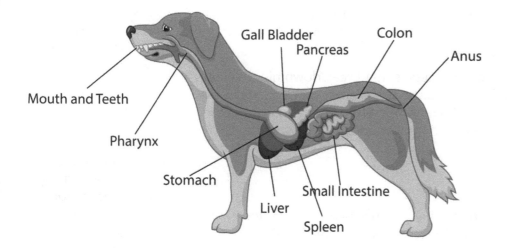

Figure 4.5 The organs of the digestive system

Dentition

An animal's digestive system begins with food entering the mouth (sometimes with the help of the tongue) where it is broken down mechanically by the teeth and chemically by saliva. Different animals have different arrangements of teeth, according to the food they have evolved to eat. Generally speaking this depends on whether they are carnivores, herbivores or omnivores. Carnivores only eat meat and have sharp canine teeth and incisors (front teeth). Herbivores are vegetarian and do not need to tear off flesh so they do not have prominent canine teeth – instead they have developed broad and flat molar teeth with which to grind up plants. Omnivores eat both plants and animals, and their teeth display characteristics of both carnivores and herbivores.

Enzymes

The tongue transmits taste sensations to the brain which causes the salivary glands to produce saliva. There are a number of chemicals called enzymes in saliva which begin the breakdown of food: amylase which breaks down carbohydrates and lingual lipase which begins to break down fats. There is also lysozyme, which acts as an antiseptic.

From the mouth food travels down the oesophagus and into the stomach. In non-ruminants there is only one stomach. It is where the major breakdown of food occurs, by mechanical and chemical means. The stomach produces gastric acid, which is very strongly acidic. This acid affects the structure of proteins in food, exposing the chemical bonds. The stomach secretes a number of enzymes to continue the digestion of food:

- the enzyme pepsin which can break proteins down into constituent amino acids
- gastric lipase which continues to break down fats

At the same time these chemical reactions are taking place, the stomach muscles contract in order to churn up the food and move it along to the small intestine.

Catabolism refers to metabolic processes that break down biomolecules. Digestion is a catabolic process because the process breaks down food into its constituent molecules. (Anabolism refers to metabolic processes that build larger biomolecules from smaller ones, e.g.the creation of proteins from amino acids).

Absorption of nutrients

By the time it leaves the stomach, the food has been broken down into a substance called chyme, and it enters the small intestine. The chyme is broken down into very small nutrient particles which can be absorbed into the cells of the small intestine and from there into the bloodstream. To help do this some further enzymes are released:

- maltase converts maltose into glucose
- sucrase converts sucrose into glucose and fructose
- lactase converts lactose into glucose and galactose
- erepsin breaks peptides into their constituent amino acids

At the end of the small intestine most of the nutrients have been removed and the chyme becomes semi-solid and passes into the large intestine. No digestive enzymes are produced in the large intestine. From there water and any remaining nutrients are absorbed, leaving faeces which are then compacted and eventually passed out through

Jargon Buster

dentition the arrangement and type of teeth

catabolism when the body breaks down biomolecules into simpler molecules.

anabolism when the body builds larger biomolecules from smaller ones

enzyme a particular kind of protein that speeds up chemical reactions; enzymes are critical to the chemical breakdown of food.

acids chemicals with a pH number of less than 7; acids with very low pH are corrosive.

alkalis chemicals with a pH number higher than 7; alkalis with a very high pH are also corrosive

pH a measurement scale, from 1-14, of how acidic or alkaline something is; a chemical that is neither acidic nor alkaline is known as neutral and has a pH of 7; water is an example of a neutral chemical

neutralise when an acid and alkaline of opposite pH are brought together they will neutralise each other i.e. the resulting substance will have a pH of 7.

defecation via the anus.

The large intestine contains many different bacteria that perform many different functions. One is the production of vitamin K, another is the stimulation of the immune system for effect against pathogens.

Acid and alkaline secretions

The chyme from the stomach is highly acidic and would cause damage the small intestine if left untreated. Two alkaline substances are secreted in order to netruralise the acids.

The first is bile, secreted by the liver and stored in the gallbladder. As well as neutralising chyme it also helps break up fats for later digestion.

The second is pancreatic juice, secreted by the pancreas and released as food moves from the stomach into the small intestine. It contains bicarbonate, another alkaline substance that acts to neutralise the stomach acids along with bile. In addition, pancreatic juice contains further digestive enzymes:

- pancreatic lipase for the continued breakdown of fats

- amylase for the continued breakdown of carbohydrates

- elastase, trypsin, chymotrypsin and carboxypeptidase for the continued breakdown of proteins

Study tip
You do not need to know the names of the different enzymes

Hindgut fermenters

Many monogastric animals are not very good at digesting the carbohydrates present in cellulose. However some animals, known as hindgut fermenters, are almost as efficient as digesting cellulose as ruminants. They do this through a process of fermentation, by relying on bacteria that live in the large intestine. The enzyme that is required to break down cellulose is produced by bacteria and not by the animal's own body. The way in which these bacteria break down is much the same as that for ruminants, and is outlined on the next page.

Some hindgut fermenters e.g. rabbits and guinea pigs make two attempts to digest their food – the second time is through eating their own faeces. This is known as coprophagy. Faeces that have only passed through their digestive system once still contain many valuable nutrients and are quite different to faeces that have passed through a second time. In some ways it is a similar process to the way ruminants regurgitate cud and digest it again (see below). Biologically speaking, it means rabbits are efficient at extracting as many nutrients as possible from food.

Hindgut fermenters include:

- rodents

- horses

- rabbits.

Ruminants

Digestive system organs and microbial organisms

The key organs of the ruminant system are:

- the tongue

- the salivary glands

- the gastrointestinal tract consisting of:

  * the mouth

  * the oesophagus

  * the four-compartment stomach consisting of rumen, reticulum, omasum, abomasum

  * the small intestine

  * the large intestine, including the caecum

- the pancreas

- the liver

- the gallbladder

The tongue is used to direct food into the mouth and roll it around. Digestion begins with the brief mechanical action of chewing. The food is mixed with saliva and quickly swallowed. However the saliva contains no enzymes.

Swallowed food is passed from the oesophagus into the rumen, the first part of the stomach. The rumen is a container where plant material sits until it has been sufficiently broken down. As with hindgut fermenters, ruminants lack the enzymes to break down complex carbohydrates present in plants (i.e. cellulose) and rely on symbiotic bacteria, present in the rumen, to produce the necessary enzymes. These enzymes break down cellulose into volatile fatty acids – mainly acetic acid (more commonly known as vinegar). This process is known as bacterial fermentation. The fats are absorbed through the wall of the rumen and reticulum (see below) and into the bloodstream, and are the main source of energy for ruminants.

The rumen is relatively large and plant material can sit there for quite a long time, which allows the enzymes produced by the microbes to fully break down the cellulose. A by-product of the process is methane, which is expelled through eructation (also known as belching!). An animal who is unable to expel methane - for instance because they cannot stand up – will become bloated and can even die.

The reticulum is separated from the rumen by a muscle fold and is so similar to it in structure, that they are sometime considered together – known as the recticulorumen. Taken together these two compartments also act to mix up the foodstuff. The reticulum has a honeycomb 'filter'

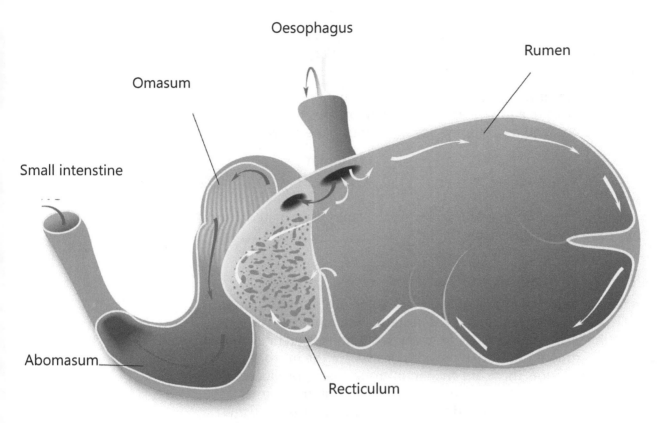

Oesophagus

Rumen

Omasum

Small intenstine

Abomasum

Recticulum

Figure 4.6 The ruminant digestive system - four-compartment stomach

that stops larger particles from entering the next part of the stomach. Instead, these particles are sent back to the rumen for further digestions, or back up the oesophagus as partially digested food that needs further chewing. This substance is known as cud (and is where the phrase 'chewing the cud' comes from). Animals spend more time chewing cud than eating food in the first place. The rumen eventually obtains fatty acids from the cellulose plant material, along with gases – carbon dioxide and methane.

Once food has been sufficiently digested it is passed from the reticulum to the third compartment of the stomach, the omasum. This compartment is where water from the food is absorbed and can also filter out any remaining particles of food that are too big to pass into the final compartment.

The final compartment is called the abomasum and is in some senses the 'actual' stomach, in that it performs the function of the stomach that we are familiar with in monogastric animals. In the same way as for monogastric animals, hydrochloric acid and a range of enzymes are secreted in the abomasum that allows fat, protein and carbohydrates to be extracted. Symbiotic bacteria are also digested as a source of protein – indeed, this is the main source of protein for ruminants and hindgut fermenters (except for horses).

As with monogastric animals, after the stomach the foodstuff enters the small intestine where most of the nutrient absorption takes place. The pancreas secretes pancreatic juice and, along with bile from the gallbladder, this reduces acidity. After that is the large intestine, where

> **Jargon Buster**
> rumen, reticulum, omasum, abomasum the four compartments of a ruminant's stomach

absorption of water and any remaining nutrients takes place.

The caecum is a pouch that sits between the small intestine and the large intestine. There are bacteria present that continue to ferment the foodstuff to obtain further energy from it.

The liver has many important functions but, as with monogastric animals, it produces bile as well as controlling hormones that control enzyme secretions, and as a storage site for various minerals and vitamins.

Dentition

As herbivores, ruminants' teeth are adapted to eating plant material and thus they have no upper incisors.

Partition of protein in the rumen

Protein can be digested in one of two ways. Some protein is known as Rumen Degradable Protein, and it is digested in the rumen by microbes. This digestion yields amino acids, from which ammonia, and ultimately nitrogen, are extracted. Nitrogen provides growth for the microbes, and so this process ensures there are enough microbes being produced. Some of those microbes in the rumen will pass through the normal digestive system, and those that do are killed and then broken down into amino acids in the abomasum and absorbed in the small intestine. Thus the microbes themselves are a source of protein.

The alternative source of protein for the animal is via direct digestion in the abomasum of Undegradable Dietary Protein – i.e. protein that microbes are unable to break down in the rumen.

The most common ruminants are:

- sheep
- cattle
- goat

Quiz Questions

1 Explain what role each of the following organs perform when it comes to digestion in monogastric animals: a) the mouth, b) the oesophagus, c) the stomach, d) the small intestine, e) the large intestine.

2 Explain what role each of the following organs perform when it comes to digestion in ruminants: a) the mouth, b) the rumen, c) the omasum, d) the abomasum.

3 What does 'partition of protein' in ruminants refer to?

4 What is a hindgut fermenter and given an example of one.

5 Give two examples of ruminants.

6 What is the purpose of a) the mucosa, b) the serosa.

LO2 Understand nutritional values and properties of different food types

2.1 Nutritional components of food, suitability of different types of fresh and prepared foods and the considerations when developing a feeding plan

In this topic you will learn about the nutritional content of different types of food, including:

- fresh and natural food

- processed food

- nutritional needs and typical diets

- considerations for a feeding plan.

Nutritional content of food

The nutrients that are described in Learning Outcome 1 of this unit are normally obtained by animals through their diet. Different food types have different quantities of nutrients. A balanced diet for an animal will ensure that they receive nutrients in the correct quantities. However, because each species has different nutritional requirements a balanced diet for one species is not necessarily a balanced diet for another. Animals of the same species can also have different nutritional requirements, depending on age, lifestyle, medical conditions and so on.

Understanding the nutritional requirements of food is a key part of putting together a feeding plan for a particular animal.

Fresh and natural food

This catch-all term really means food that has not been processed in any way. It includes fruit, vegetables, grasses and meat.

- Fruit and vegetables: low in fat, low in salt, low in calories; good source of vitamins, minerals and fibre.

- Grass and foraged food: only animals that can break down cellulose, namely hindgut fermenters and ruminants, find any nutritional benefit to eating grass and other plant material. For those animals grass provides energy from carbohydrates, as well as protein, fibre and minerals. Grass is a natural source of food for a number of livestock animals, as well as rabbits, and given a choice animals would normally prefer grass over hay. As a food source grass is also much cheaper than processed food. However there are reasons why hay might be a preferred food source (see below).

- Meat: carnivores require meat for some essential nutrients – for instance we have seen that cats are carnivores and must eat meat for an essential fatty acid and an amimo acid. Meat is an excellent source of protein but contains no carbohydrates. It is a source of energy however because of the relatively high fat content. Red meat and pork have high levels of saturated fat whereas lean cuts of chicken have low levels of fat. Red meat is a good source of zinc and iron, and vitamins B2, B6, B12.

- Live food: sometimes animals that are still alive are fed to carnivores or omnivores. Examples include mealworms for birds, crickets for certain reptiles and mice for snakes. However, this practice is controversial because the nutrients that the predators are fed do not depend on eating live animals. There is a responsibility on those working with animals to care for all of their welfare needs – and that includes the animals that are being used as food. Live food might be considered as 'natural' by some people but you must remember that any animal that is not in the wild is not in a 'natural' environment.

	Fruit and vegetables	Grass and foraged food	Meat
Protein	High levels for beans, peas, leafy green vegetables	Yes for ruminants and hindgut fermenters.	Very high
Carbohydrate	Low	Yes for ruminants and hindgut fermenters.	None
Fat	Low	Low	High for red meat
Vitamins	High levels	Vitamin A, B, C, E.	Good source of B-vitamins. Liver is a good source of vitamin A, D, E K and B-12.
Minerals	High level	Calcium, phosphorous, magnesium, iodine, zinc.	Meat is a good source of iron and zinc. Chicken is a good source of selenium.

Fresh food does not stay fresh for long and there is a limited timeframe when it is suitable for eating. Fresh food that is past its best may taste bad or develop mould which would pose a health hazard. There is also a significant risk of food poisoning from food that has gone off, particularly meat.

Prepared and processed food

Animal food is commercially available in processed forms. These include:

- Dry food: this tends to be in the form of pellets or biscuits and is therefore convenient to store as it keeps for a long time. It also tends to be better for animals' teeth than wet food. By its very nature there is less water present in dry food, so particular care must be taken to provide an adequate supply of water. Dry food will tend to contain more carbohydrates, derived from cereals, than wet food.

- For livestock a common dry food is hay, which is essentially dried grass. In the drying process the grass will of course lose moisture but also loses nutrients, and can be harder to digest. Hay is more expensive than grass, but it keeps for much longer and is often used when fresh grass is not available, for instance in winter.

- Wet food: this tends to be available in sealed containers, which means that is also easy to store – but it will spoil once opened and the food is served. Wet food tends to be more expensive than dry food. With fewer carbohydrates and therefore more protein and fat, animals may prefer the taste and smell of wet food.

- Semi-moist: this tends to be like the dry biscuits but with greater water content. These may contain more sugar so care should be taken for animals with diabetes.

- Processed food is available for all animals and, depending on the species, might also include a mixture of seeds, grains, nuts and dried fruit.

Prepared and processed food will keep for much longer than fresh food and is often therefore more convenient. However even processed food can develop mould if not stored correctly, in which case it would also pose a health risk.

Poor storage can also put the food – fresh or processed – at risk of contamination. For instance, the presence of food can attract wild animals which may lead to contamination with faeces or urine. This would be a significant health risk.

Typical diets

Commercially available animal food is regulated in the UK, and manufacturers follow the European Pet Food Industry Federation (FEDIAF) nutritional guidelines. These guidelines are very detailed and define the minimum nutrient content for different species.

Pet food labels are also regulated, so that consumers can be sure that what they are buying is suitable for their animal. Animal food that is labelled as 'Complete' means that the food is guaranteed to include all of the required nutrients for a particular animal with a particular lifestyle. For instance food that is 'complete' for an adult dog will not be complete for a puppy or a pregnant bitch. The size of the animal is also important, particularly with dogs because they can range from very small to very big.

Pet food can be 'wet' (normally in cans) or 'dry'. There are pros and cons for both, but both can contain a complete range of nutrients.

There is a wealth of further information available on the Pet Food Manufacturers' Association website www.pfma.org.uk

Similarly, pre-prepared mixed feeds are also available for farmed animals, designed for that species at a particular life stage and lifestyle, e.g. calf pellets, sheep nuts.

It is of course possible to construct bespoke diets for animals too, based on their specific nutrient requirements. It is not a simple task to ensure all minerals and vitamins are included, particularly as the presence of some vitamins inhibits the effectiveness of others. However it is important to know and understand the different dietary requirements of common animals.

Dogs

As we have seen, there are essential amino acids that animals must obtain from protein in their diet. About 18-25% of a dog's diet should come from protein. The source of protein can be animal or vegetable – as long as the vegetarian sources include all of the essential amino acids. However animal sources tend to be easier to digest. Dogs do also use protein as a source of energy.

Similarly, the supply of essential fatty acids can come from animal or vegetarian sources. Fat should account for at least 5-10% of the diet.

Dogs do not need carbohydrates because they can make glucose from protein sources, and so carbohydrate is not an essential nutrient for a dog. However, if carbohydrates are present in the diet then dogs can obtain a proportion of their energy needs from them. Carbohydrates can come from things like oats, grain, corn and wheat.

The minimum requirements of vitamins and minerals is detailed and too complicated to list here. Further information can be found in the following places:

https://www.petcoach.co/article/protein-requirements-for-good-nutrition/

https://www.msdvetmanual.com/management-and-nutrition/nutrition-small-animals/nutritional-requirements-and-related-diseases-of-small-animals

Cats

As has already been discussed, cats are carnivores because they cannot synthesise the amino acid taurine – they can only obtain it from animal products. Therefore they will need a diet that includes some animal-derived products. Cats need a lot more protein than a dog – about 25%-35% of their diet should be made up from protein.

Fat should make up at least 9% of a cat's diet and, again, the essential fatty acid arachidonic acid can only be found in animal sources.

As with dogs, cats have no dietary need for carbohydrates as they can derive all of their energy needs from protein and fat. However including some carbohydrates is not harmful and indeed most commercially available cat food contain them.

Other animals

Nutritional requirements and diet are different for different animals and these details can change depending on the lifetstyle or role of the animal – for instance, dairy cows have different dietary needs than beef cows.

There is not enough space to cover the needs of all animals here but this useful resource summarises requirements across a range of species:

https://www.msdvetmanual.com/management-and-nutrition

Considerations when developing a feeding plan

When developing a feeding plan you need to think about the following:

- What are the nutritional requirements of an average adult?

- How will these requirements need to be changed if the animal is:

  * newly-born

  * not fully grown

  * old

  * very active – perhaps a working or racing animal

  * very inactive – perhaps due to an injury or condition

  * pregnant

  * overweight / underweight

  * any other factors that might deviate from the average adult.

- How will the food be stored and delivered?

(Do note that commercial products may be available that take into account the factors above for some species.)

Once you have an understanding of the specific nutritional needs of the animal(s) you are considering, then you can devise a feeding plan that takes account of them by using the nutritional information associated with different foodstuff, whether that is fresh or prepared.

Quiz Questions

1 Give two examples of fresh food.

2 Is meat high or low in a) protein, b) carbohydrate, c) fat?

3 What are the pros and cons of wet versus dry pet food?

4 Which animal needs more protein, a dog or a cat?

5 List two considerations when developing a feeding plan.

LO3 Understand the feeding requirements of animals at different life stages

3.1 Calculate rations for animal diets

In this topic you will learn how to calculate the nutritional requirements for an individual animal so you are able to specify the following in a feeding plan:

- feed items and ingredients

- the amount of food and its energy value

- quality of the foodstuff

- a comparison of the nutritional values of wet and dry diets

- the gross energy (GE), digestible energy (DE) and metabolisable energy (ME)

- resting energy requirements (RER and basal metabolic rate (BMR)

- calculations of the rations of different foods to meet nutritional requirements.

As we have seen, nutritional requirements are different according to species, size and lifestyle/life stage of each animal. This must all be taken into account.

As well as the correct balance of food, the correct quantity of food must be served each day. This is known as the daily ration. If the ration of food is too high then the animal may become obese. If the ration of food is too small then the animal may become emaciated.

Feed items and ingredients

A feeding plan must include details of:

- Fresh water provision – clean water is essential so the plan must describe how an animal can access it, in a way that is appropriate for its circumstances. For instance, an elderly animal may not be able to reach up or bend down.

- How will food be delivered to the animals?

- What ingredients will make up the diet? Is the food fresh or dry?

- Will supplements be needed for some or all animals being fed?

- How will the food be stored?

Jargon Buster

calorie a unit of energy. Confusingly 'Calorie' is often used in nutrition but the scientifically accurate term is kilocalorie or kcal. We will use 'kcal' when performing calculations but use the nutritional term calorie when discussing the final result.

metabolisable energy the energy in food that the body can extract and use for bodily processes.

obese overweight

emaciated underweight

Calculate the energy content

Pet food labels list the 'analytic constituents' as a percentage. Typical constituents include protein, fat, ash and fibre. Each of these contains a certain amount of metabolisable energy (see page 89). Typical values are:

- protein: 3.5 kcal per gram

- fat: 8.5 kcal per gram

- carbohydrate: 3.5 kcal per gram

- fibre: 0 kcal per gram

- ash: 0 kcal per gram

- moisture: 0 kcal per gram

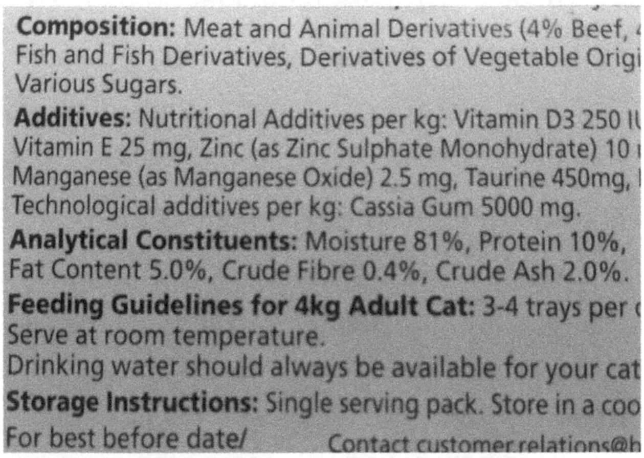

Composition: Meat and Animal Derivatives (4% Beef, Fish and Fish Derivatives, Derivatives of Vegetable Origi Various Sugars.
Additives: Nutritional Additives per kg: Vitamin D3 250 I Vitamin E 25 mg, Zinc (as Zinc Sulphate Monohydrate) 10 Manganese (as Manganese Oxide) 2.5 mg, Taurine 450mg, Technological additives per kg: Cassia Gum 5000 mg.
Analytical Constituents: Moisture 81%, Protein 10%, Fat Content 5.0%, Crude Fibre 0.4%, Crude Ash 2.0%.
Feeding Guidelines for 4kg Adult Cat: 3-4 trays per Serve at room temperature.
Drinking water should always be available for your cat
Storage Instructions: Single serving pack. Store in a coo
For best before date/   Contact customer relations@h

Figure 4.7 Pet food label

So, to calculate the amount of energy per gram in pet food you need to take the following steps:

1. Check whether 'carbohydrate' has been listed in the analytical constituents. If not, then you need to add up all of the other constituents to work out how much carbohydrate is present.

2. You can calculate the number of kcals per 100 gram of food by using the figures above for protein, fat and carbohydrate.

3. Once you know how many kcals there are per 100 gram of food, you can calculate the energy per serving of food. For instance if you served 70 grams of food, then you would multiply the kcals per gram by 0.70.

Worked example

A pet food label has the following information:

Analytical constituents: crude protein 23%, fat 13%, moisture 10%, ash 6.5%, fibre 2.5%, calcium 1.4%, phosphorous 1.1%.

Step 1.

Notice that the percentage of carbohydrate has not been listed. Therefore we need to calculate it. We do this by adding up the percentage of all of the listed ingredients:

> 23% + 13% + 10% + 6.5% + 2.5% +1.4% + 1.1% = 57.5%

We have accounted for 57.5% of the contents, so the remainder must be carbohydrates, i.e.

> % of carbohydrates   = 100% - 57.5%
>
> = 42.5%.

Step 2.

Now we calculate the kcal for each ingredient for a 100g serving, using the table above:

> protein: 23% of 100g = 23g of protein

3.5 kcal of energy per gram of protein, so there are 3.5 x 23 = 80.5 kcal of energy.

fat: 13% of 100g = 13g of fat

8.5 kcal of energy per gram of fat, so there are 8.5 x 13 = 110.5 kcal of energy.

Carbohydrate: 42.5% of 100g = 42.5 g

3.5 kcal of energy per gram of carbohydrate, so there are 3.5 x 42.5 = **148.75 kcal** of energy.

Total energy content of 100g of this food = 80.5 + 110.5 + 148.75

= **339.75 kcal**.

Using the nutritional units, this is 339.75 Calories.

Step 3

Now you know how much energy there is per 100g you can calculate the energy for any serving size.

For instance if you served 150g then the energy would be:

150/100 x 339.75

= 509.63 kcal

= **510 Calories**

Or a 70g serving would be:

70/100 x 339.75

= 237.83 kcal

= **238 Calories** (rounding up and using the nutritional units).

Assess the quality of food stuffs

For commercially available feed the manufacturer will provide detailed and accurate nutritional information. However, for home-made diets or ingredients, for farmers who let livestock graze, or who grow crops for feeding animals, some method of assessing nutrition will be needed.

The quality of food is really a measure of how nutritionally valuable it is; a low quality feed, for instance, would have low levels of essential nutrients and might require supplements, or need to be fed in large volumes. Conversely a high quality feed would provide all of the necessary nutrients. Unsurprisingly, a low quality feed would normally be cheaper than a high quality one.

Nutritional information is available online for common foodstuffs and crops. A good resource to consider is www.feedipedia.org

Such websites can be used as a guide when assessing home-made diets. However the exact nutritional composition of a particular crop will depend on the growing conditions, soil, climate etc. So, as with any feeding plan, it is important that careful monitoring of the plan takes place, to make sure that its impact on animal behaviour or output is observed.

More sophisticated methods of establishing the nutritional components of a particular batch of crops or food can be undertaken in laboratories. These include various chemical analyses, studies on digestibility and NIR (near infrared) spectrometry techniques. However these are more expensive options.

Compare the nutritional values of wet and dry diets

At first glance it appears that dry and wet food have quite different percentages of nutritional ingredients. However the percentages on food labels are not comparing like with like, because of the difference in moisture content between the two. To accurately compare the nutritional values you must assess only the dry ingredients. You do this as follows:

Worked example

Let's take the analytical constituents of a dry food label to be:

crude protein 30%, fat 15%, moisture 10%, ash 5%, fibre 3%, calcium 1.5%, phosphorous 1.1%.

Because 10% of the dry food is moisture, which has no nutritional content at all, this means 90% is the dry food value. All of the nutritional content is in this 90%. So, we want to work out how how much protein, fat etc. there is compared to this 90%. We do this as follows:

% of ingredient in 'dry part' of food = % of ingredient on the label / (100 – moisture content %)

Remember that both wet and dry food has a 'dry part' - and this is what we are referring to here.

So, % of crude protein in dry part of food is

= % of crude protein on the label / (100 – moisture content %)

= 30% / (100 – 10)%

= 30% / 90%

= **33%**

and % of fat in 'dry part' of food is calculated using

= % of fat on the label / (100 – moisture content %)

= 15% / 90%

= **16.7%**

This method can be extended for any ingredients that are listed. Notice that the % of dry foodstuff is equal to 100% minus the percentage of moisture content.

For wet food, typical values of protein, fat and moisture might be:

crude protein 8%, fat 6%, moisture 75%.

Using the same method as above,

% of ingredient in 'dry part' of food = % of ingredient on the label / (100 – moisture content %)

So, % of crude protein in dry part of food is

= % of crude protein on the label / (100 – moisture content %)

= 8% / (100-75)%

= 8% / 25%

= **32%**

and % of fat in 'dry part' of food is

= % of fat on the label / (100 – moisture content %)

= 6% / (100-75)%

= 6% / 25%

= **24%**

You can now compare these percentages with those calculated above for dry food. Now that you are comparing the food on the same basis you will notice that the percentage of protein and fat is much more similar than the food labels would appear to suggest. Only the last two rows are a direct comparison of the nutritional values across wet and dry food.

Summary of results

From the last worked example we have the following results:

	Protein %	Fat %
Dry food label percentage	30	15
Wet food label percentage	8	6
Dry part of dry food %	33	16.7
Dry part of wet food %	32	24

Gross energy (GE), digestible energy (DE) metabolisable energy (ME)

Energy is a widely-used term but when used scientifically it has a precise definition, which is 'the capacity to do work'. The Gross Energy (GE) of foodstuff, then, is is a measure of how much chemical energy it contains that can be converted into other forms.

When an animal eats food, as we have seen, not all of it is digested. The food that passes through the body undigested still contains chemical energy which the body has not been able to convert. Therefore the energy the body has been able to digest (Digestible Energy) equals the gross energy of the food minus the energy that passed out of the body in stools.

Digestible Energy (DE) = GE – energy in faeces

Some of the digestible energy is converted by the body but used in the production of urine and gases. So, the total Metabolisable Energy (ME) equals the Digestible Energy minus the energy used to produce urine and gas:

Metabolisable Energy (ME) = DE – energy producing urine and gases

It is the metabolisable energy of foodstuff that can meet an animal's daily energy need.

Jargon Buster

Gross Energy (GE) the total chemical energy in food that can be converted into other forms

Digestible Energy (DE) the amount of GE that the body is actually able to digest

Resting energy requirement (RER) and Basal Metabolic Rate (BMR)

In order to work out how much food an animal needs, you need to understand their individual energy requirements.

The Basal Metabolic Rate (BMR) is a measure of how much energy is needed to run the body's basic functions – such as breathing. Measurement of BMR is under very strict conditions and does not account for any movement or even digestion of food. So, a more useful measure is the Resting Energy Requirement (RER), which describes how much energy is needed for an animal at rest. RER will always be larger than BMR.

You can estimate the RER in Calories for cats and dogs by multiplying their bodyweight in kg by 30, and then adding 70:

RER = (weight in kg x 30) + 70

Jargon Buster

Basal Metabolic Rate (BMR) the amount of energy required to run the basic bodily functions and processes

Resting Energy Rate (RER) the amount of energy required for an animal at rest. RER is always larger than BMR

Worked example

For example, for a dog of 25kg, their RER is:

RER = (25kg x 30) + 70

RER = 750 + 70

= 820 Calories.

This value of 820 Calories is the energy needed for a 25kg dog that is completely inactive. You can multiply the RER by different numbers to estimate for different lifestyles and conditions – see the next section.

Calculate rations of different foods to meet requirements.

Now that you know how to calculate the energy in a portion of food, and you also know how to estimate the energy requirement of an animal, you can work out how much of a particular food to feed an animal each day.

Worked example

Use the figures we have calculated previously, i.e. you are creating a feeding plan for a dog with an estimated daily energy requirement of 820 calories. You want to know how much of the food we have looked at to feed him. For that food, we calculated that a 100g serving contained 340 calories. So, to work how many servings of 100g you should serve a day:

daily serving = energy requirement of animal / energy supplied by 100g of foodstuff

= 820 / 340 calories

= 2.41 servings of 100g per day.

A simpler way of putting it is that the dog will need 241 g of this food per day – almost a quarter of a kilogram.

Average voluntary food intake

Another way that you can calculate ration size is through average voluntary food intake for a particular species. These are often expressed in kg of dry food as a percentage of overall body weight. (Because the calculation is based on dry food, a further calculation would be needed to work out the wet food mass.)

Worked example

For sheep the average voluntary food intake (AVI) in kg is around 2.5% of body weight. You can calculate the dry food ration size for sheep as follows:

Ration size = AVI/100 x animal's weight

For a sheep weighing 65kg the calculation is:

ration size = 2.5/100 x 65

= 0.025 x 65

= 1.63 kg

For a sheep weighing 43kg:

ration size = 2.5/100 x 43

= 0.025 x 43

= **1.08kg**

If the animal was being fed wet food with a 75% moisture content, then the amount of wet food needed would be:

= 1.08 / (1-0.75)

= 1.08 / 0.25

= **4.32 kg**

The quoted figure for AVI will be relevant to an animal at a particular life stage and with a particular lifestyle. You should bear this in mind when applying this formula.

All of the calculations above are approximations because each animal is different. You may find that a particular animal does not lose or gain weight by eating a little more or less than calculated, and is otherwise healthy considering their age, lifestyle and condition. Monitoring the effects of a feeding plan will ensure that you can adjust ration sizes as appropriate for the animal(s) you are feeding.

Quiz Questions

1 Calculate the total amount of energy contained in serving of pet food with the following analytical constituents: crude protein 25%, fat 11%, moisture 8%, ash 6%, fibre 3.5%, calcium 1.8%, phosphorous 1.3%.

2 Compare the following dry and wet food by calculating the percentage of protein and fat on the same basis, i.e as percentage of the dry food. DRY: crude protein 28%, fat 17%, moisture 9%, ash 6%, fibre 3%, calcium 1.5%, phosphorous 1.1%. WET: crude protein 10%, fat 7%, moisture 73%.

3 Define: gross energy (GE), digestible energy (DE) metabolisable energy (ME)

4 Define Basal Metabolic Rate (BMR) and Resting Energy Rate (RER).

5 Calculate the RER for a dog with a mass of 12kg.

6 Calculate the ration of food for the dog in question 5 eating the food from question 1.

3.2 Dietary requirements for different life stages and conditions, and how these influence the development of a feeding plan

In this topic you will learn how to calculate the energy requirements of animals at different life stages and in different conditions, including:

- juvenile

- adult

- geriatric

- breeding/pregnancy/lactation

- working

- obesity

- anorexic

- specialist veterinary diets eg diabetes, laminitis

- recuperation.

You will also learn how to choose an appropriate diet to meet those requirements.

Animals at different life stages, with different lifestyles or particular medical conditions, will have different nutritional needs than an 'average adult'. In particular their energy needs will be quite different.

For a dog, the following factors can be used as a guideline, to correct the resting energy requirement as calculated in section 3.1, for the following conditions:

- Weight loss for an average adult: 1 x RER

- Normal activity adult: 1.8 x RER

- Normal activity neutered adult: 1.6 x RER

- Sick animal: 1 x RER

- Light working dog: 2 x RER

- Moderate working dog: 3 x RER

- Heavy working dog: 4 x RER

- Early pregnancy: 1.8 x RER

- Late pregnancy: 3 x RER

- Nursing mother: 4-6 x RER depending on the number of pups

- Puppy (1 to 4 months): 3 x RER
  - Puppy (4 to 12 months): 2 X RER

Source: http://www.mpcoftexas.com/public/Caloric_Guide_for_Dogs.cfm

For a cat:

- Weight loss for average adult: 0.8-1 x RER
- Normal activity adult: 1.4 x RER
- Normal activity neutered adult: 1.2 x RER
- Sick animal: 1 x RER
- Pregnancy: 2.3 x RER
- Nursing mother: 2.6 x RER
- Kitten: 2.4 x RER

Source: http://petnutritionalliance.org/

So, if our 25kg dog on page 89 is non-working and doing a normal amount of exercise, then you will need to multiply the RER by 1.8:

> = 1.8 x RER
>
> = 1.8 x 820
>
> = **1476 calories per day.**

In general the following guidelines apply:

- Juvenile – need more energy for growth.
- Adult – the benchmark energy value that all the others should compare to.
- Geriatric – older animals normally need less energy as they are less active.
- Breeding/pregnancy/lactation - more energy is required by pregnant animals and new mothers.
- Working - more energy is required – the amount does depend on how intense the work is.
- Obesity – less energy is required for animals who are overweight, in order that they use some body fat for energy instead.
- Anorexic – underweight animals need more energy.
- Specialist veterinary diets e.g. diabetes, laminitis – different conditions have different requirements. For diabetes, it is important that the animal is not underweight or overweight, so the energy intake needs adjusting if so. The aim of a diabetic diet is to regulate blood sugar, which means reducing fat and increasing fibre and complex carbohydrates at the expense of simple sugars. Horses with

laminitis also need to reduce intake of simple sugars and ensure they have enough high quality protein.

- Recuperation – animals who are sick normally need less energy than normal.

Quiz Questions

1 Do the following animals normally require more or less energy than an average adult of the same species and breed?

    a Geriatric
    b Working
    c Young
    d Pregnant
    e Obsese.

LO4 Plan, monitor, record and evaluate diets and feeding regimes for animals

4.1 Design a feeding plan

In this topic you will learn how to design a feeding plan, and create a record card, for a selected species, life stage and condition. The plan will include:

- fresh water and its delivery

- choice of diet

- appropriate quantities of food

- frequencies of delivering food

- methods of food delivery

- alternatives to the plan dependent on food availability.

Fresh water and its delivery

As we know water is essential for animals, so a feeding plan must explain how fresh, clean water will be made available for all animals at all times.

Choice of diet and appropriate quantities of food

As we have seen in LO3 the choice of diet depends on a number of factors. Your plan should detail what that diet should contain and what quantity of food should be served on a daily basis. This would include details of fresh or prepared food, and any food supplements that need to be added.

Frequencies of delivering food

Food may need delivering at certain times of the day, or more frequently than just once. Your plan should direct exactly when and how often.

Methods of food delivery

The plan must consider how food will be delivered to the animals. If there are mutliple animals then it must have provisions in place to ensure all animal have equal access. Consideration must be given to animals who have special requirements or conditions that might make feeding difficult. If there is unlikely to be enough room around one feeding station then multiple stations must be included.

Food can be delivered to animals in different ways and the plan must cover this. When delivering food there is an opportunity to think of creative enrichment activities in which an animal could be stimulated at the same time.

In the wild animals can spend most of their time finding and eating food. In contrast, a typical pet spends very little time eating because it is (almost literally) handed to them on a plate. Delivering food in a way that can stimulate an animal will help prevent boredom and lengthen meal times, which may prevent over-eating.

Ideas to enrich feeding times for pets include placing food in more than one location and hiding treats that the animal will discover at some point during the day. There are also puzzle feeders available, where the animal is rewarded with food once they have figured out how the feeder works. However, food must not be so well hidden that it stops the animal from eating and fresh water does need to easily available at all times.

Alternatives to the plan

It may be that food in the plan is not always available, particularly if the diet is made up from fresh food. You should detail potential alternatives that would provide the same nutritional and energy requirements.

Record card

Once a feeding plan is being implemented it is very important that the following are recorded each day:

Jargon Buster
turbidity cloudiness

- Consumption of food and water.

- Health status.

- Animal behaviour.

- Frequency and turbidity of urination.

- Frequency and consistency of defecation.

Recording all of this information will allow any potential health or behavioural issues to be spotted early. It will also inform any amendments to the feeding plan that may be required for specific animals.

4.2 Understand how to monitor, record and evaluate the effectiveness of a feeding plan

In this topic you will apply what you have learned by creating and evaluating a feeding plan over a period of 4 – 6 weeks.

For this learning outcome you need to put into practice the feeding plan that you have designed in 4.1. You will then need to monitor the implementation of the plan, record what happens using your record card, and then evaluate the effectiveness of the plan.

You will need to ensure that your record card observations are accurate. You can then use those results to evaluate the effectiveness of your feeding plan. The kind of things you will need to consider as part of your monitoring and evaluation are:

- Health status: Have their been any positive or negative impacts of the plan? Were the aims of the plan met with regard to health? Were there any unintended consequences of the plan with regard to the animal's health?

- Condition: Is the animal putting on weight? Is it losing weight? What does its coat, fur, skin etc. look like? Are they in good condition?

- Quantities: How much food and water is the animal consuming? Given the calculations about energy requirements, is that enough to provide a balanced diet? Aside from energy, are there enough other essential nutrients for the lifestyle and conditions of the animal in question?

- Cost: What are the actual costs of feeding the animal? How does that compare to the budget you had in your feeding plan? Could you find alternatives food types that might have an impact on costs? Is the amount that it is costing to feed the animal reasonable for the size and species?

You will need to talk to your lecturer about which animal you select to monitor. It may be one that is kept at your college or institution, or it may be one kept elsewhere. The main consideration is that your feeding plan can be put in place, and you can have regular access to it for 4-6 weeks to observe and record.

Quiz Questions

1 Name three things that you need to include in your feeding plan.

2 List three observations you should record on a daily basis.

3 How would you evaluate your feeding plan with regard to effect on health?

END OF UNIT QUESTIONS

1. a) List all of the major nutrients required for a balanced diet.   (6 marks)

_____

2 Describe the chemical structure of the amino acid glycine.   (3 marks)

_____

_____

_____

3. State **one** function for each of the following parts of the   (4 marks)
digestive system of a dog.

a) tongue

b) stomach

c) small intestine

d) large intestine

_____

_____

_____

4. Give **two** examples of animals that are hindgut fermenters.
                                                                (2 marks)

_____

5 Describe the digestive processes that take place in a ruminant's (5 marks)
stomach.

_____

_____

6 State **four** things you need to consider when developing a
feeding plan for a household cat.   (4 mark)

_____

_____

_____

7. Explain why a farmer may choose to feed dairy cows pre-prepared animal feed.   (4 marks)

_____

_____

_____

_____

8. a) Define the gross energy (GE) of foodstuff.t   (1 mark)

_____

_____

b) Define digestible energy (DE).   (1 mark)

_____

_____

c) Define metabolisable energy (ME).   (1 mark)

_____

_____

9. A cow has a dry matter average voluntary intake of 3% of body weight. Calculate the average voluntary intake of a cow weighing:

a) 600 kg (1)   (2 marks)

b) 450 kg (1)   (2 marks)

_____

_____

_____

_____

_____

_____

10. Evaluate **three** factors that should be considered in the feeding plan for a pregnant pig.   (3 marks)

_____

_____

_____

Unit 305 Animal Behaviour and Communication

LO1 Understand behaviour patterns in animals

1.1 Analysis of natural and atypical animal behaviour

In this topic you will learn about natural and atypical behaviour in animals, to include:

- foraging

- hunting

- sleeping

- social behaviour

- grooming

- courtship

- territorial

- hyperactivity

- excessive inactivity

- displacement behaviour

- stereotypic behaviours.

Domesticated animals or pets do not suddenly lose the instincts associated with their wild ancestors and cousins. These instincts dictate much of their behaviour, so it is important that you understand what is typical, and what is not, for a range of species.

Foraging

In the wild, animals need to find food. This is known as foraging. Behaviour associated with foraging for food includes:

- sniffing around for sources of food

- eating leftovers – whether or not the food was meant as leftovers!

- eating food that grows in the wild, including fruit and grass

- eating faeces if it contains some nutritional content
- hoarding of food that has been found
- territorial behaviour based on guarding food – see below.

Hunting

Carnivores and omnivores have developed strategies to seek out other animals as sources of food and then to overpower them. Hunters in the wild may roam around in order to find prey, may sit still in the same spot and wait for prey to come to them, or they may combine elements of both behaviours.

Animals in captivity may demonstrate elements of this hunting behaviour:

- Dogs often have a desire to chase after other animals (or even cars!).
- Vigorous shaking of a toy, cloth or stick in a dog's mouth simulates the way a dog might kill prey.
- Herding behaviour in sheepdogs derives from chasing and rounding up prey.
- Sniffer dogs' abilities are derived from the desire to seek out and track prey.
- Domestic cats will stalk and sometimes kill animals such as birds and rodents.
- Cats will also employ a sit-and-wait tactic.
- Hunters often adopt a 'point and freeze' stance when 'prey' is detected.
- Play-fighting (either with other animals or humans) simulates the behaviour needed when subduing prey.

Sleeping

- Dogs will sleep for hours at a time across different times of the day, and may spend around 12 hours asleep each day – although this depends on species, age and the individual animal.
- Rodents and rabbits are often referred to as nocturnal i.e. they sleep during the day and wake at night. However in actual fact many of them are actually crepuscular, which means they are most active at dawn and dusk, and sleep at other times.
- Cats can sleep from 12-16 hours a day, although that tends to be a light sleep so they can react to any perceived threat. They are most active at dawn and dusk i.e. crepuscular.
- Whilst birds can sleep normally they are also able to sleep with only one half of the brain at a time. This allows them to keep one eye open and alert whilst partly asleep. If the right-hand part of the brain is asleep then the left eye can be kept open and vice versa.

Jargon Buster
crepuscular animals that are active at dawn and dusk

- Horses sleep standing up, for about three hours per day.

  - Cows and sheep will sleep lying down if they are comfortable and safe in their surroundings, for about four hours per day.

  - Pigs sleep lying down for about 8 hours per day.

> **Activity**
>
> Find out about the typical sleeping patterns of the particular species of animal you are studying.

Social behaviour

Social behaviour refers to the way in which animals interact with each other. These interactions may be for a range of different reasons, such as finding food, shelter or a mate. Some behaviours may be shared amongst entire classes of animals – for instance mammals – whereas others may be species-specific. Even within a species different breeds may have different traits and tendencies, and of course individual animals will also have their own tendencies too.

- Social units may consist of a full group (e.g. wolf packs or a pride of lions), a pair of adults of the opposite sex (such as is the case with many bird species), or solitary adults (e.g. various big cats in the wild).

- For feral cats the formation of a social group is due to the perceived benefit of sharing food and resources, and safety in numbers. With domestic cats, whilst resources such as food are not in short supply and they are not normally in any danger, and whilst they do have a tendency towards solitary behaviour, they can still form social groups. When domestic cats are in the same social group you will see them grooming each other and sleeping together. If they are not part of the same social group then multiple cats in one house may regard each other as tolerated rivals. Alternatively they may be aggressive with each other. Cats can also be aggressive with other cats who do not live with them who appear in their territory (e.g. the garden).

- Dogs are social animals, which means that they do not like to be by themselves and seek out the company of familiar dogs or humans. This trait means that they need to be able to understand social signals. In practice this means that dogs learn to predict how other dogs and humans will behave in certain situations and then form their social bonds based on these predictions. In this sense a dog is truly a part of the family.

- These ideas displace the common belief that relationships with and between dogs is about 'dominance'. This came from research into wolf-pack behaviour in the 1960s and the assumption that dogs were domesticated wolves. However the original ideas about wolf behaviour have been replaced, as further research has revealed that wolves live in family units that are not trying to dominate each other – there is far more cooperation than was previously assumed. It has also been recognised that dogs' behaviour cannot be assumed to mimic that of wolves. As a result the theory of dominance as the key tool to explain dogs' social behaviour has been widely abandoned.

- Dogs will behave differently with strange dogs compared to familiar dogs, as each tries to establish how the other dog will react. Strange dogs will approach other with some caution and each may have some associations or inherent behavioural traits that will lead them to be be friendly, playful, aggressive, fearful etc. But regardless, each dog will try to predict the other's behaviour and react in a way that it thinks is the most appropriate.

- Typical social behaviour of dogs includes: barking, to warn other members of the family about intruders or potential danger; play-fighting; smelling each other to establish mood and behaviour; sleeping together; greeting returning members of the family.

- Other animals that like the company of their species include: horses, donkeys, cows, pigs, sheep, goats, chickens, gerbils, mice and rats.

- Common solitary animals include hamsters and most reptiles.

Grooming

Grooming animals will use their tongue, mouth, beaks and paws. It serves several purposes in animals:

- It's the primary way that many animals keep clean, through the removal of dirt, parasites, faeces and urine.

- Social animals often groom each other. Although it can be helpful for hard-to-reach spots, social grooming provides a way for animals to build social bonds between each other and reinforce the social structures that exist between the group.

- Just as with massages for humans, the act of touch can be pleasurable and relaxing, which can reduce stress levels in the animal and provide other benefits to health.

- Animals may rub against an object, such as a post or a wall, as part of their grooming routine.

- Dogs will lick and use their teeth to remove dirt and debris but will also roll around in grass, dust, carpet or against furniture as part of their grooming routine.

- Cats will lick themselves directly and lick their paws in order to clean themselves all over. It also helps them to regulate body temperature and promote blood circulation.

Courtship

Unlike humans, many female mammals have oestrous cycles when they are 'on heat', and are only sexually active during this time. Courtship typically occurs only when the female is on heat, because hormonal changes means she secretes pheromones and behaves in a way that signals to the male she is sexually receptive. General signs of heat in a female are a swollen, reddened vulva and mucous discharge. Species-specific courtship behaviour includes:

Jargon Buster

oestrous the time in a female reproductive cycle when they are fertile and ready to mate, or 'on heat'

perineum the area between the anus and genital area

Dogs

- Mounting and thrusting behaviour from males.

- Females may back into males.

- Females will 'flag' their tail – lift it out of the way.

- Males may follow females around and be more aggressive with other males.

- Males will try and smell or lick the female's perineum.

- Males and females may display playful behaviour towards each other e.g. the play bow.

Cats

- Male and female cats will call out to try and find available mates.

- Males will spray urine to both find females and warn other males off.

- The male and female cats will spend some time touching and licking each other.

Horses

- Tail is erect and adopts the same position as when urinating.

- Actively seeks out other horses.

- Mares stand still with hindquarters facing a stallion.

- The flehmen response – when a horse bears its upper lips and inhales in order to breathe in and detect pheromones.

Sheep

- Ewe finds a ram and stays near it – may separate from the flock.

- Ewes form a harem, raising and wagging their tails.

- Ram displays flehmen response (as with horses), may lift front leg onto a ewe and vocalise.

Cows

- Raised, twitching tail, with arched back.

- Seeks a bull through bellowing.

- Cows may attempt to mount other cows.

Rabbits

Rabbits do not have an oestrous cycle – instead they ovulate once they have mated.

Territorial

In the wild an animal, or group of animals, often try to establish claim or access to a particular area or patch of land. By doing so they may guarantee access to resources they need. This instinct is strong in some animals and will be displayed in pets or domesticated animals too.

- Urine is often used by animals to mark their territory. This communicates information to other animals, including the area is occupied. However this information is not simply a 'keep out' sign – for instance cats often have overlapping areas, and use scents to establish how long since another cat was present in order to avoid confrontations.

- Other scents can also be used for the same purpose, though may communicate different things. You can see this when cats rub their head or body on inanimate objects (or you!).

- They may also leave physical signs of their presence – bite or claw marks.

- Animals may also mark their territory through sound – by howling, hissing or growling.

- Dogs will often growl or bark at strangers who are near to, or have been permitted into, their territory.

- Animals may become possessive about certain toys, their food bowl or bed, and display some tense, aggressive behaviour if they are interfered with.

- For dogs, their human owners may form part of their territory – and therefore may display some of the behaviour above if they feel 'their' humans are under threat.

Hyperactivity

Also known as hyperkinesis, animals can display behaviour that is similar to ADHD (Attention Deficit Hyperactivity Deficiency) in humans. There is something of grey area between a highly energetic animal and one with hyperactivity but some symptoms are:

- chasing own tail
- spinning around and around
- constant movement
- short attention span, that stops the animal from concentrating on one task
- impulsive and easily distracted
- destructive behaviour.

Jargon Buster
hyperkinesis another term for hyperactivity

There are a number of reasons why animals might be hyperactive:

- Environment – chaotic surroundings and lack of structure/routine will exacerbate any animal's tendency towards hyperactivity.

- For pets, small children can excite young animals which may affect their behaviour as an adult. The relationship between children and animals should always, of course, be carefully monitored.

- For sociable animals such as dogs, lack of contact with humans and/or other dogs can cause them to behave in an over-simulated fashion when they do have contact.

- Lack of exercise can also play a part – dogs will need a certain amount of exercise each day to provide structure and help 'burn off' some energy.

- Diet is important for all aspects of animals' health, and hyperactivity can be a symptom of poor diet.

- Genetics – each animal is different of course, and some will be more prone to hyperactivity than others. However environment plays an equally important part, particularly when young, and therefore the ideas above can help animals who are prone to the condition.

- An underlying medical issue such as a malfunctioning thryroid can also lead to hyperactivity.

Excessive inactivity

The opposite problem from hyperactivity is abnormal inactivity. What is considered normal depends on the species and breed of animal, and whether they are wild or in captivity. (Captive animals tend to be less active than their wild counterparts). Common symptoms are:

- prolonged periods of inactivity, either sitting, standing or lying down

- lack of response to stimuli

- body language that suggests they are withdrawn

- less vocal than normal.

When humans suffer depression, symptoms can include withdrawal into themselves and a lack of desire to interact with the rest of the world. There is some evidence to suggest that for animals inactivity is linked to their mental state brought on by their environment.

- Sociable animals need stimulation from their companions, so a lack of opportunities for social interaction will affect them. If such animals are starved of this when they are young, this may affect them in their adult life.

- Boredom. As well as social interaction, animals need mental stimulation to prevent them becoming bored. This might be in the form of games or puzzles, or by encouraging foraging for food.

- Another possible reason for inactivity is the animal is ill or in bad health. This may be caused by poor diet or poor living conditions.

Displacement behaviour

This can occur if an animal is torn between two contradictory urges (e.g. curiosity about a new object and fear of the same object), or is somehow prevented from doing something they really want to. Instead they perform a seemingly meaningless and unrelated act, such as:

- scratching,

- self-grooming,

- touching themselves.

This behaviour can be a signifier of the stress level of an animal, though that might not always be true. These acts are similar to human behaviour in stressful situations, such as scratching, wringing hands, nervous coughing etc.

Stereotypic behaviour

Stereotypy means the repetition of a movement or action for no particular reason. In animals this would include:

- pacing up and down, or round and round

- rocking back and forth

- repeated vocalisations

- tossing the head up and down

- moving a limb back and forth

- repeated biting or tongue movements

- excessive grooming.

Stereotypic behaviours are often linked to stress and mental well-being. These are often caused by:

- a lack of opportunity to forage for food

- poor diet (can lead to oral stereotypy)

- lack of space, relative to natural behaviour in the wild

- growing up in a stressful environment.

Stereotypic behaviour is not observed in wild animals and therefore are normally a sign that something is wrong with the captive environment.

> **Jargon Buster**
> stereotypic behaviour repetitive actions or movement without a particular aim or goal

Quiz Questions

1 Give two examples of stereotypic behaviour.

2 Give one example of displacement behaviour.

3 Give two examples of hyperactive behaviour.

4 What behaviour might indicate excessive inactivity?

5 How do animals mark their territory?

6 Describe two functions that grooming performs.

7 When are cats at their most active?

8 What is the technical term for an animal 'on heat'?

1.2 Causes of atypical behaviour in animals

In this topic you will learn about the causes of atypical behaviour, including:

- **confinement**

- **unsuitable environment**

- **inappropriate social grouping.**

Atypical behaviour is often caused by one or more of the following:

Confinement

Confinement of any animal is unnatural. However accommodating a small animal with a limited natural territory is easier than for a large animal that roams over a wide area in the wild. The density of animals is also a factor – i.e. even a large area might be inadequate if there are too many animals, or the animals are naturally solitary. This a potential problem in zoos and farms. So-called 'battery' or 'factory' farms, where individual animals have exceedingly limited space, are very likely to see displays of abnormal behaviour. In the EU and UK, by law caged battery hens must be housed in enriched cages with a certain amount of space, a separate area to lay down in and must be able to stretch their wings and have a place to perch.

For companion animals a natural roamer such as a cat is likely to display some abnormal behaviour if confined indoors.

Unsuitable environment

Any environment that is not clean, dry and warm, with access to adequate food and water, and somewhere to go the toilet, is likely to induce stress. In addition, opportunities for exercise, play and intellectual stimulation are also necessary for many species. Deficiencies in any of these can lead to atypical behaviour.

It goes without saying that the environment should also be free of hazards

Inappropriate social grouping

Different species have different requirements regarding other animals. Getting this wrong can lead to aggression and/or mental stress. Examples of inappropriate groups include:

- naturally sociable animals being kept alone

- naturally solitary animals being kept in groups

- forcing together individual animals who, whilst sociable, are in different social groups

- incorrect social structures within social groups, e.g. adolescents maturing into adults that would have left the group in the wild, introduction of new animals that upset the established hierarchies

- it may sometimes be inappropriate for different breeds to live together

- removal of family members, for animals who establish such groups

- competing males and/or females during mating periods.

Close proximity to other species may also cause serious stress – particular for predator and prey species. In that case stress may be induced in both the predator and the prey.

Quiz Questions

1 Why might confinement be a problem for a cat?

2 Give one example of an unsuitable environment.

3 Give two examples of inappropriate social grouping.

1.3 Behaviour of captive or domestic animal and wild counterpart

In this topic you will learn about the differences in behaviours between wild animals and their captive or domesticated counterpart e.g.:

- wolf and dog

- wolf in the wild and in the zoo

- wild cat and domestic cat.

Behaviour of wild animal	Behaviour of domestic or captive animal
Wolf • Even hand-reared wolves do not make strong social bonds with humans. • Wolves live in a family unit with a breeding pair. • Pups will begin to explore after around two weeks. • Wolves are wary of novel situations and people/animals. • Wolves do not look at humans for visual cues. • Wolves regurgitate food for pups. • Wolves rarely bark but do howl.	**Dog** • Makes very strong attachments with humans • Feral dogs in a pack do not stay in a family unit, and may breed within and without the group. • Pups will begin to explore after around four weeks • Socialised dogs can cope with novel situations and people/animals • Dogs will make eye contact with humans and glean cues from their body language • Dogs rarely regurgitate food. • Dogs are more likely to bark than howl.
Wolf • Will display fear or aggression towards humans. • In the wild the pack's territories are large and varied which encourages exploration. • The family hierarchy of the pack is dynamic and allowed to develop naturally. • There is no alpha wolf – the packs consist of parent figures and extended family.	**Wolf in zoo** • Socialised wolves (i.e. those that have been reared in the zoo) are less likely to be fearful of humans, and show some interest in them. They may still show aggression however. • With less space, or uninteresting layouts, captive wolves are less likely to explore. Packs in captivity are not necessarily families and therefore do not develop in the same way as in the wild. This can lead to aggression, particularly to those low down in the hierarchy. • The idea of an 'alpha wolf' came from studies of unrelated wolves in packs in captivity.

Wild cat	Domestic cat
• Largely solitary. • Large territory, with a core area where they feed and sleep. • Uses various scents and markings to communicate and mark territory. • Does not rely on facial expressions for communication. • Spends a great deal of time hunting for food. • Prefers to run to safety rather than fight if in danger. • Careful, private and hygienic in their toileting habits. • Prefers running water • Likes an elevated sleeping place.	• Willing to share space with human owners and can form social groups. • Smaller territory but with a core area. • Uses various scents and markings to mark territory. Does not rely on facial expressions for communication. • Has a strong urge to hunt, even though they do not need to for food. • Prefers to run rather than fight, and need places they can hide. • Careful, private and hygienic in their toileting habits. • Likes to have access to high places where they can see all of their surroundings.

Quiz Questions

1 List two ways in which a wolf's behaviour differs from a dog and explain why the behaviour is different.

2 List two ways in which a captive wolf's behaviour differs from a wild wolf and explain why the behaviour is different.

3 List two ways in which a cat's behaviour is similar to a wild cat.

LO3 Understand the factors influencing behaviour

Animals in the wild exhibit behaviour that is partly due to their genetic code, inherited from their parents, and partly due to things they have experienced since birth. These two factors are often referred to as nature and nurture, and both have a large impact on the behavioural characteristics of individual animals.

3.1 Evolution of behaviour

In this topic you will learn how evolution informs animal behaviour, including:

- **link between environment and behaviour**

- **heredity of behaviour**

- **differences between development and evolution**

- **Darwinian Theory**

- **domestication.**

Link between environment and behaviour – adaptation and competition for resources

The environment can influence an animal's behaviour in two different ways.

In the wild, a stable environment over many, many generations will influence the evolution of a species in such a way that they become perfectly adapted to the conditions. For instance, the camel is perfectly adapted to living in the desert as it can survive without water for many days by storing fat reserves in its hump. When it does find water a camel will drink a large volume at a time.

There are many examples of animal species who have have evolved over time to become perfectly adapted to their environment. This happened because their ancestors lived in the same environment for a very long time.

The environment can also cause an animal to change behaviour over its own lifetime. For instance, there is a great annual migration of wildebeest across the Serengeti plains in Africa that is driven by a dry/rainy season. If the climate changed and the pasture did not dry out then the wildebeest would not embark on their epic journey each year.

Animals are often in competition with each other, from the same and different species, for food and resources. Changes to competition e.g.

113

a new species encroaching onto territory, might lead to changes in an animal's behaviour, such as increased aggression or a change in feeding/ hunting habits.

Domesticated animals are also influenced by their environment – for instance, animals enclosed by electrified fences on farms will learn to not approach the perimeter of the field.

It must be be noted that any changes in animal behaviour over their lifetime are still limited by their genetic code. Limits to their mental or physical capacity, due to their genes, might mean they are unable to change their behaviour.

Heredity of behaviour

Heredity is defined as the passing on of traits from parents to offspring. They can be physical or mental traits. The mechanism for heredity is through the passing on of genetic material; however the ideas of heredity were understood before anyone had discovered genes.

There are two aspects to heredity of behaviour. In the first case, animals display some behaviour that they have not learned and is completely 'hard-wired' into them. This behaviour is inherited and passes from one generation to the next and is known as innate behaviour. Further discussion of innate behaviour is on page 118.

Most behaviour, however, is due to a combination of learning and genes. So in this second case, behaviour may need to be learned but an animal can only do so if it has the necessary genes.

For instance, certain breeds of dogs are more disposed towards hunting than others. That is because certain genes that are present in 'hunting breeds' such as spaniels. However they still need to learn how to hunt. Other breeds of dog, however intelligent, will never learn to become hunting dogs because they do not have the necessary predisposition, due to their genetic make-up. Meanwhile an animal such as a rabbit can never be taught to hunt because no species of rabbit has the necessary genes to enable such behaviour.

So, to summarise: heredity influences some behaviour directly, and also provides limits on physical and mental characteristics that determine what an animal can learn and therefore how it behaves.

Differences between development and evolution

Evolution is a process whereby a species' heritable characteristics change over many generations. The mechanism for evolution is described by Darwinian Theory (below).

Development consists of the changes that an animal undergoes during its lifetime, beginning at conception and ending at death. These changes include things like the way in which an animal grows, from a newborn to an adolescent, and on to a full adult, and includes all physical, mental and behavioural characteristics.

Development depends on evolution because each species can only

Jargon Buster
heredity the passing on of traits from parents to offspring

innate behaviour an action that an animal has not learned

develop in ways that its genetic code allows – for instance, even though it has the intellectual capacity to problem-solve, a dolphin will never be able to perform a task such as opening a bottle because it doesn't have fingers and thumbs. The evolutionary history of dolphins has provided a limit that each animal's development cannot overcome. In this way evolution defines the parameters within which development takes place.

However whilst animals within a species will normally display very similar traits, development is different for each individual animal because genes only define the potential - the environment and experiences of the animal ultimately define whether that potential is explored or not. For instance, all elephants have the genetic potential to grow to be large animals; but a young elephant with malnutrition will not grow as large as a young elephant that has a good diet.

Darwinian Theory

In the 19th century Charles Darwin developed the theory of evolution by natural selection. It says that:

- animals within a species display a range of different heritable characteristics

- there is competition for resources which means that some animals in a species will not survive long enough to reproduce

- animals with characteristics that are better suited to their environment are more likely to survive and pass them on to offspring

- those successful characteristics are therefore passed on to the next generation, whilst less successful characteristics, that led to animals dying, are less likely to be passed on.

As this pattern repeats over time the helpful characteristic becomes more common in the species. Over many generations this eventually becomes common to the entire species – and means that the species has adapted to its environment.

The subsequent discovery of genes explained exactly how characteristics were passed from generation to generation.

Examples of animal characteristics that are explained by Darwinian Theory include:

- Darwin studied finches on the Galapagos Islands off the coast of South America. They had different beaks to the finches on the mainland. Finches on the islands had developed a wide range of different beak shapes according to the food they ate – large beaks for cracking nuts and small beaks for eating insects. Darwin realised that the finches were perfectly adapted to the environment and competition on each island.

- Peppered moths were originally pale but the species changed to a darker colour during the industrial revolution in Britain, in order to blend in more easily with pollution-stained buildings.

- Insects developing resistance to insecticides (e.g. moths and DDT), bacteria developing resistance to antibiotics (e.g. the 'superbug' MRSA.)

Darwin's ideas were controversial at the time because they challenged the idea that humans were separate from animals. However there is now overwhelming evidence from a range of sources, including an extensive fossil record, to support Darwin. It is by far the best evidence-based explanation we have for how life on Earth has developed.

Domestication

Domesticated animals are not just tame wild animals; they have genetic differences from their wild counterparts, or ancestors, that include a natural tolerance or friendliness towards humans. The first animal to be domesticated was the dog, but humans went on to domesticate a number of animals for different reasons: e.g. cows, sheep and chickens for food, horses and donkeys for work, and cats for other mutual benefits (in the case of the cat, killing vermin like mice and rats).

It is widely acknowledged that animals need to have certain natural traits in order to be domesticated. This means that many species of animals can't be domesticated. The traits include things such as:

- Can be fed easily – for instance, it was relatively easy to ensure grazing animals such as cows could be provided with food.

- Temperament – animals that scare easily or are naturally aggressive are not normally suitable candidates for domestication – although note there is something of an exception with regard to wolves and dogs.

- A social structure amongst the species that predisposes them to relationships with humans.

- Will breed in relatively small spaces. Animals that require a large territory for breeding will not be successfully domesticated.

Over time animals that humans kept in captivity developed genetic differences which led to the truly domesticated species that we know today. Domestication of animals (and plants) allowed humans to stop being hunter-gatherers and instead begin farming. (As an aside, it is interesting to reflect on how this in turn led to the development of more sophisticated human cultures and civilisations, leading to technology and the complex societies that exist today).

Dogs

Dogs and the grey wolf share a common wolf ancestor. It is commonly accepted that at some point – possibly as long as 40,000 years ago – some of those wolves learned to live with humans. These animals eventually split off, in an evolutionary sense, from wild wolves to become the first ancestors of dogs. It is not clear exactly where in the world this split first happened – various theories suggest Europe or Asia, or both. And it may have happened more than once. The first recorded remains of a 'modern' dog buried with a human date from 14,000 years ago, in Germany. This demonstrates that dogs had been domesticated by this point.

Given that wild wolves would have posed a threat to human it interesting to consider how domestication happened. There are two theories: the first is that humans tamed some wolves, possibly by adopting wolf pups, and purposely pursued their subsequent domestication. The second, more widely accepted theory, is that some of the less aggressive and 'friendliest' wolves approached humans, probably because the humans provided a source of food. With limited food resources, the friendlier wolves would have gained an advantage over other wolves and subsequent generations would have inherited this trait. This second theory is called self-domestication.

Humans were able to use domesticated wolves for work, such as hunting and guarding, and hence the relationship was mutually beneficial.

These early dogs were probably still semi-wild, living in and around settlements and feeding off scraps. But the seeds were sown for the deep and long-lasting partnership that dogs and humans have had ever since. Once humans began to breed dogs, then 'natural selection' was no longer a mechanism for their evolution – instead there was artificial selection, with dogs selected for breeding because of their physical and behavioural characteristics. This has led to the wide range of dog breeds, many of which bear little resemblance to their wolf cousins.

Quiz Questions

1 Explain how the environment affects animal behaviour in terms of a) adaptation, b) competition for resources.

2 What does heredity mean?

3 Explain the difference between evolution and heredity.

4 Outline Darwinian theory.

5 Explain how dogs might have evolved from wild wolves.

3.2 Development of behaviour

In this topic you will learn how development informs animal behaviour, including:

• difference between instinctive and learned behaviour

• trial and error

• observational learning

• parental or social teaching

• cultural behaviour.

117

Difference between instinctive and learned behaviour

As discussed previously, animals display some behaviour that has not been learned and is completely 'hard-wired' into them. This behaviour is known as instinctive. Examples of instinctive behaviour include:

- Moths are attracted to sources of lights and will always fly towards them.

- Newborn mammals automatically suckle milk from their mother.

- The kneading action of a kitten on their mother.

- All reflexes – such as pulling away from touching something hot – are examples of innate behaviour that does not need to be learned.

- Sleeping patterns of animals.

An instinct may still require some external stimulus to trigger the reaction.

Some animal behaviour may appear to be instinctive but in actual fact has been learned at an early age. For instance, ducklings following their mother around appears to be instinctual. However experiments have shown that ducklings will follow the first moving object it sees after it is born – even if that is a human. So their instinctive behaviour is simply to follow but they normally learn to follow their mother.

Behaviour can also be a mixture of instinctive and learned. For instance many animals can walk not long after birth. Whist the ability to walk might be innate, they will also learn how to walk more effectively with time, and eventually run.

Trial and error

Animals can learn through trial and error at any age. Learning takes place through doing, and then assessing the outcome. If the outcome is positive then they are likely to repeat the behaviour but if the outcome was negative then they are less likely to repeat it. There have been many experiments on rats in which there is a maze to navigate in order to receive some food. The rats quickly learn the quickest route to the food, and then remember it the next time they are put into the maze.

Much training of dogs relies on their ability to learn through trial and error, often through positively rewarding desired behaviour with treats.

Observational learning

Trial and error is a useful way of learning in order to solve problems but it can be very risky if the activity is potentially dangerous because the 'error' might result in injury or death. However, animals can also learn by watching other animals and copying them.

Animals learn a lot from watching their parents, peers or other animals of their species. Examples of observational learning include:

- Young predators such as tiger cubs learn to hunt by watching their parents.

  - Primates observe and copy the foraging behaviour of other members of their social group.

  - Young birds learn to fly by watching their parents.

  - Song birds also learn the full detail of their species' songs by observation.

  - Dogs who are unsure of water watch other dogs jump in and start swimming.

  - The marsh warbler is a song bird that is influenced by other species of birds that it hears. Thus each bird has a different song.

In observational learning, the learners may acquire new behaviour by watching animals who are not actively trying to teach them.

Parental or social teaching

In other scenarios experienced animals will actively teach inexperienced animals, which normally requires more interaction that simply observing. For instance, parents may gently punish their offspring for undesired behaviour to discourage it.

Some examples of parental teaching include:

- meerkats will teach their young how to eat prey that is potentially dangerous, such as scorpions, by introducing them to incapacitated animals first

- big cats such as cheetahs will bring prey to younger animals, to help teach them how to hunt

- birds called pied babblers use a particular call when delivering food to their young, that they later exploit to encourage the young to leave the nest

- ants will lead other ants to food

- killer whales teach their young to intentionally beach themselves on land to catch certain prey.

Cultural behaviour

Culture means the adoption of particular behaviour across groups. There is some evidence that animals may adopt and transmit new or different behaviour in this way. Whilst the learning itself takes place through observational learning and social teaching, the behaviour becomes commonplace across large groups.

A good example that could be explained by culture is that of certain birds learning to peck at and open milk bottles which used to be left outside people's houses. In doing this they were able to drink the cream at the top of the bottle. This behaviour was widespread in the UK when milk bottles were a common sight outside. There is some disagreement as to whether cultural learning really took place but there is some evidence for it.

There is some evidence that the same species of some songbirds have different 'dialects' according to their geographical location which would suggest a cultural aspect to their behaviour.

Some research on wild rats in Israel suggested that their tendency to strip pine cones before eating was transmitted only amongst that particular group, and rats from elsewhere who were not familiar with pine cones did not display the same behaviour. This strongly suggested that there was a cultural aspect to the way in which rats are able to learn.

There is still much research needed to provide evidence that a wide range of species exhibit cultural aspects to their behaviour but there are many who believe that it is widespread.

Quiz Questions

1 Give some examples of instinctive behaviour.

2 Explain what is meant by 'trial and error'.

3 How do some birds learn by observation?

4 How might hunting skills be passed on to the next generation for predators?

5 What is cultural learning? Give a well-quoted example.

3.3 Factors influencing behaviour

In this topic you will learn about internal and external factors that influence behaviour, including:

- hormones

- fixed action patterns

- other animals

- seasonal variation such as food availability, daylight, weather.

Hormones

Hormones are chemical messages that are sent around the body to change certain characteristics and behaviours. They are fundamental to the major body systems because they regulate and control them. They are involved in a huge range of physical processes.

Hormones are created in a range of glands that make up the endocrine

Jargon Buster
endocrine system a series of glands and chemical signals that regulate the actions of numerous organs within the body

120

system and then sent around the body via circulatory systems such as the bloodstream.

Whilst hormones control bodily processes, evolution has ensured that they also influence behaviour related to that process. For instance, the sex hormones testosterone and oestrogen are responsible for the growth of sperm and eggs but are also responsible for mating behaviour in adults. Mating behaviour is thus aligned to the periods when sperm or eggs are at their prime and therefore when fertilisation is more likely to take place.

Hormones have an influence in:

- levels of aggression

- mating behaviour

- parental behavioural

- social behaviour – because responding to other animals in appropriate ways is important for reproductive success.

Examples of hormones that influence behaviour include:

- Testosterone can lead to aggressive behaviour, e.g. the highest levels of aggression in male deer occurs in autumn when testosterone levels are at their highest; castration normally reduces levels of aggression in males across species.

- Progesterone is thought to be involved in maternal behaviour, e.g. in rats males and females who aren't mothers or pregnant have a tendency to avoid baby rats, whereas mothers are very protective of them, coinciding with decreased levels of progesterone, which allows increased levels of another hormone called proclatin.

- Oestrogen is linked to the behaviours associated with being in oestrus/heat.

It is important to note that hormones influence behaviour but behaviour also influences the production of hormones. It is also important to note that whilst hormones influence behaviour they do not uniquely control behaviour. A male will not begin a mating ritual when there are no females around, regardless of how much testosterone is being produced.

Fixed action patterns

Fixed action patterns are behaviours that are hard-wired into animals. They require some external stimulus, but once begun the behaviour tends to continue on through a sequence of 'action patterns' regardless of any further stimulus from the environment. A particular stimulus for a particular species almost always results in the same predictable behaviour for a fixed action pattern.

Examples of fixed action patterns in animals include:

- Mating rituals and dances in certain species, such as peacocks, are triggered by the presence of the opposite sex. The rituals themselves are the same across animals.

- Herring gull chick instinctively peck at a red spot on their parents' beaks, which triggers the parents to feed them. The instinct to peck is triggered by the red spot, and chicks will peck at any red spot they see, regardless of whether it is on a beak or indeed a gull.

- Male stickleback fish will become aggressive with other males during mating season. The males of the species have a red underside. However, introducing other red objects into their environment triggers an attack from the male fish. Therefore 'seeing red' is the trigger for this aggressive behaviour.

- Domestic cats display fixed action hunting patterns when they are stimulated by small moving objects even if they are not prey – this might be demonstrated through stalking or swiping with a paw.

Other animals

The presence of other animals can have a dramatic effect on animal behaviour.

If the other animal is of the same species, then they can affect behaviour due to:

- sexual attraction

- competition for a mate

- competition for resources or territory.

If the other animal is of a different species then they can affect behaviour due to:

- fear of an unknown species

- fear of a known predator species

- competition for resources or territory.

The instinctual behavioural response to other animals may be overridden by learned responses. For instance, it may be quite possible for domesticated animals of different species to live in close proximity if they have been exposed to each other since birth. There are limits to how far a natural instinct can be suppressed however - it is unlikely that a cat and a mouse can live happily together.

Seasonal variation

The different seasons also have an affect on animal behaviour. This might be spring, summer, autumn and winter but also includes wet and dry seasons in other parts of the world. They can affect behaviour in a number of ways:

Food availability

Plants tend to stop growing in winter and during rainy seasons which can lead to food shortages for animals that feed on them and their predators. As a result animal behaviour can change in the following ways:

- **Hibernation**. With food sources scarce in winter, some animals adopt a low energy sleep-like state for a period of time that can last several months in some species. In this state bodily functions such as heart rate and breathing slow down, and the animal is able to survive for longer periods without food.

- Some animals also **hoard food** before the winter comes, hiding it away to be retrieved when food is very scarce. Hoarding behaviour is triggered by the change in seasons.

- Another way of coping with decreased food availability is to simply **travel** to find food elsewhere. This means covering large distances and is not an option for many animals. Some species of birds, such as swallows, 'fly south for the winter' for precisely this reason and cover thousands of miles. Other mass migrations, such as with the wildebeest in Africa, are in response to the lack of resources available in the dry season.

- **Territorial behaviour increases** in some species as food becomes scarcer because each group needs to protect the diminishing resources in its territory.

- **Breeding**. Many animals have adapted to make sure that they do not give birth immediately before or during winter, when food is scarce and temperatures are harsher. This means that availability of food has an affect on the timing of breeding seasons.

- Scarcity of food may lead to animals becoming **less selective about their food sources**. For instance, when there is plenty of food predators will often choose the easiest prey in order to conserve energy. As food becomes more scarce, a predator may have to hunt animals that are harder to catch or more likely to put up a fight.

- Seasonal variation of food may also lead to **increased aggression** when food is scarce.

Daylight

Most animals have adapted to the regular cycle of night and day, with many hormonal and biological processes governed by it – these are known as circadian rhythms. Hours of sleep is perhaps the most obvious example of how the hours of daylight affect an animal's behaviour.

Some animals are active during the day whilst others are nocturnal and active during the night. Any change in daylight hours across seasons therefore has an impact on the hours of activity for all animals.

Daylight hours has an affect on animals with a seasonal breeding cycle. For instance, the oestrous cycle in sheep coincides with the decreasing hours of daylight; this ensure that lambs are born in spring when food is available as grass is growing again.

It should be noted that the seasonal variation of hours or daylight depends on latitude – i.e. how far north or south you are. For animals who live around the equator, there is no seasonal variation in daylight

Jargon Buster
circadian rhythm an internal clock that regulates bodily processes

hours. For animals that live in the far north or far south, there is an extreme variation – the most extreme being 24 hours of daylight and 24 hours of night at certain times of the year.

Whilst we have covered many of the changes in behaviour due to food availability, often the trigger for the changed behaviour is the change in daylight hours. This is because, unlike temperature or other factors, daylight hours change in the same way over a year and have done so for millions of years. This means that animals have evolved to use them as an indicator. As an example, whilst the reason for hibernation is the lack of food brought on by winter, the change in daylight hours can be the trigger for hibernation in some species (rather than change in temperature).

Weather

Seasonal changes in weather has a large impact on the availability of food and thus impacts on animals in that way. Daylight hours are also connected to the change in weather – as days get longer, weather tend to get warmer. But for animals that hibernate underground it is the change in temperature, rather than hours of daylight, that causes them to wake up.

For some animals living in harsh desert conditions the only way to survive the hot and dry season is to take shelter underground. This might require tunnelling and nest building at certain times of the year. A seasonal rainy season will cool things down and allow these animals to emerge from their shelter, search for food and breed.

Similarly, animals may also dig tunnels or build warmer nests to escape from cold weather. Other animals, such as emperor penguins, may have built up reserves of fat to keep warm during the extremes of the Antarctic winter.

Some animals, such as the snowshoe hare, may change the colour of their coat across the year, to camouflage themselves in snow and in order to conserve heat (as a white coat retains heat better than a darker coat).

Cold-blooded animals do not need to maintain a constant body temperature and instead ultimately reach the same temperature as the ambient temperature. They rely on the ambient temperature to drive their metabolic processes. Their activity is therefore tied very directly to the weather and how it changes over the year.

Quiz Questions

1 What is a hormone?

2 How do hormones influence behaviour and give an example?

3 What is a fixed action pattern? Give an example.

4 How might the presence of another animal influence an animal's behaviour?

5 What seasonal variations might influence a animal's behaviour?

LO4 Understand social behaviour and animal communication

4.1 Methods of communication

In this topic you will learn about the methods of communication between animals of the same and different species, including:

- vision

- hearing

- chemical

- touch.

Communication between animals is important because it provides a way for different animals to transmit information to each other. This information might be about how they feel (e.g. threatened, aggressive, calm, keen to mate) what they are about to do (e.g. attack, withdraw), or it might be information about a third party, place or object (e.g. a potential source of food, the presence of a predator).

Communication is often between animals of the same species (intraspecific) or between animals of different species (interspecific).

The behaviour of one animal can and often does have an influence on the behaviour of another through different methods of communication. Understand and predicting the behaviour of other animals is key to creating social groups that can live together and communication is at the heart of that.

Jargon Buster

intraspecific between the same species

interspecific between different species

Study tip

To remember the difference between inter- and intra, remember that intrASpecific is the SAme species

Vision

Animals (and humans) communicate how they are feeling through their body language and facial expressions. For instance, a dog can adopt a number of different postures according to how it feels (figure 5.1):

- Alert – tail up, ears forward, closed mouth, raised up on paws.

- Dominant aggressive – tail up and large, ears forward, mouth open and lips curled, baring teeth, raised hackles.

- Fearful – tail down, ears back, lowered body.

- Happy or playful – tail up or wagging, ears up, mouth open, crouching down with front paws.

Similarly, a cat will also communicate its mood and behaviour through its posture (figures 5.2):

- Alert – ears up, sat up straight, tail on the floor possibly moving slowly back and forth.

a

b

c

d

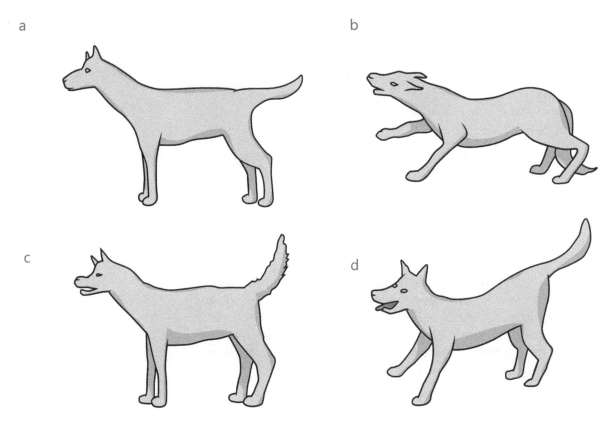

Figure 5.1 Body language of a dog: a) alert, b) fearful, c) dominant aggressive, d) happy or playful

a

b

c

d

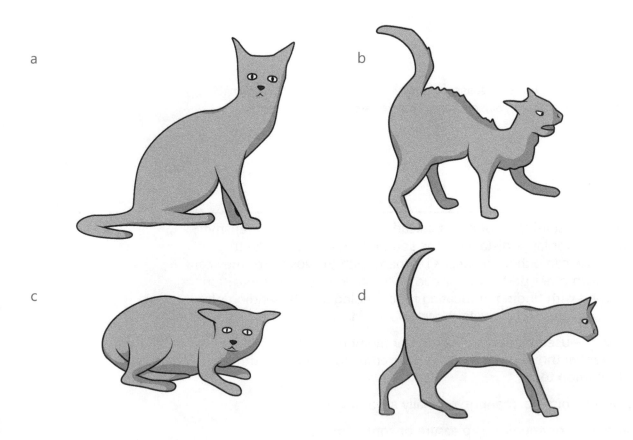

Figure 5.2 Body language of a cat: a) alert, b) aggressive, c) fearful, d) happy or playful

- Aggressive – tail up and bushy, ears down, fur stood up, arched back, mouth open.

- Fearful – crouched down, muscles tense, tail tucked away, dilated pupils.

- Happy or playful – tail up and curled, closed mouth, standing in a relaxed posture. A cat that is feeling happy and trusts you will expose its belly.

There are many more different moods that can be communicated with subtle differences in posture and movement.

There are of course differences between cats and dogs in the meaning of their body language. It is unsurprising that the two species can find it hard to interpret each other's moods and intentions and do not always get on.

Whilst humans have the most expressive faces, with a reported 27 different facial expressions, animals can also display different emotions with different expressions. Socialised animals have more expressions, and animals like dogs, cats, horses and chimpanzees have numerous different expressions. Some of the characteristics of these expressions are similar across different species, for example:

- wide eyes often demonstrate an alerted state

- piercing, hard stares often are a sign of agitation or a direct challenge

- baring teeth, unsurprisingly, is often a sign of aggression

- yawning when not tired can be a sign of stress.

Activity

Find out what body language communicates the following emotions in three animals of your choice: fear, aggression, happy/contented

Hearing

Sounds are a useful form of communication because they can transmit information over large distances. The sounds that animals make to communicate can either be vocal – i.e. made with the voice – or they can be made with other parts of their body. Much auditory communication is concerned with finding or locating food, finding a mate, fending off predators or warning off rivals. Vocal sounds include:

- barking – used by dogs to alert other members of the pack to a potential threat but is likely to be used to communicate other information too

- growling, hissing, roaring– normally a warning sound

- purring – communicates pleasure or contentment

- howling – used for a range of reasons e.g. marking territory

  - whimpering – can be associated with submission

  - singing – used by birds and whales, to define their territory and for attracting mates

  - vocalisations are often used as a method of communication between mothers and new-born offspring.

There are many other examples across lots of different species. Some, like the songs of humpback whales, are very complex and sophisticated – so sophisticated in fact that there is some evidence of differing dialects in different areas.

Non-vocal communication examples include:

- 'chirping' of crickets and grasshoppers – known as stridulation, this sound is made when crickets rub their wings together, and when a grasshopper rubs its wing with its leg

- the infamous sound of the rattlesnake, made by shaking the distinctive end of their tail

- the slap of a dolphin tail on the surface of the sea

- gorillas beating their chest.

> **Activity**
>
> Research and describe some more vocal and non-vocal auditory communication.

Chemical

All processes in an animal's body, at a fundamental level, are a series of chemical reactions; they are constantly creating and synthesising chemicals. Animals have evolved to react to certain chemicals emitted by other animals. These chemicals are known as pheromones, and each one can trigger certain behaviour in animals.

Animals give off smells other than pheromones, and these can still communicate something about the animal in question. They do this using their sense of smell (the olfactory system) and taste. Many animals have a more developed sense of smell than humans and can detect complex information from different smells.

This chemicals responsible for this method of communication are normally found in:

- urine

- faeces

- special scent glands, which causes animals to rub against objects.

Jargon Buster

auditory communication transmission of information through sounds

Jargon Buster

pheromone a chemical given off by an animal that other animals can detect through smells

olfactory system the sense of smell

Predators like sharks are also normally sensitive to the smell of blood in their prey.

Animals may leave these smells in order to

- mark boundaries of their territory

- to give a signal that they are looking for a mate

- to warn off rivals or aggressors

- to lure prey

- to point towards sources of food.

Touch

As a form of communication, touch (also known as tactile communication) is often used to provide comfort and stimulate the creation of social bonds. From an evolutionary point of view it makes sense that touch is very important for newborn mammals and birds, because the young are very vulnerable and rely on being close to their mothers for food. They take comfort in touching their mother and siblings, and mothers will often lick their young.

When social animals are adults they retain these tactile communication traits, e.g.:

- elephants are very tactile at all ages and will touch each other with all parts of their body, building communicating a fairly complex set of emotions and behaviour

- big cats, as well as domestic cats, will nuzzle and rub up against other members of their social group

- many animals, including primates, will groom each other – known as allogrooming – which helps to build and reinforce social structures, as well as various health benefits (see page 104)

Whilst most tactile communication is positive, touch can also be used to signal aggression or warn of an impending attack, generally along with other clear visual and auditory clues.

> **Jargon Buster**
> tactile touching
>
> allogrooming mutual grooming between members of the same species

Quiz Questions

1 What does intraspecific mean?

2 Give two examples of visual communication.

3 What is a pheromone and how can they be used to communicate?

4 Give some examples of aggressive auditory communication.

5 What is allogrooming and how is it useful for communication?

4.2 Formation and maintenance of social grouping

In this topic you will learn about social behaviour:

- **hierarchies**

- **maintenance of dtominance relationships through communication**

- **agonistic behaviour**

- **social bonding and affiliative behaviour**

- **altruism.**

The way that two or more animals interact with each other is known as social behaviour. Some animals are solitary whereas others are highly social, forming complex social groups.

Hierarchies

Social animals will form hierarchies that can be linear or complex. Their purpose is to allow groups to live together in relative harmony, because the hierarchy defines how one animal should behave to another. This prevents constant fighting and aggression over things like food and other resources. There may however be fighting and aggression amongst a newly formed social group, or when a new member is introduced to the social group, in order that the hierarchy is established.

All sorts of factors can play a part in why one animal is dominant over another – this includes size/weight, age, sex, breed, and certain anatomical features or displays.

Some animals form social groups with linear hierarchies. This means that there is a pecking order – quite literally, in the case of chickens who wait in turn to eat and drink:

- the top animal in the group is dominant over all other animals in the group;

- the second animal in the group dominant over all others except the top animal;

- the third animal in the group dominant over all others except the first two;

- and so on until you reach the last animal in the group, who has no dominance over any other animal and instead is submissive to all other animals in the group.

Some animals that display linear social hierarchies include:

- chickens

- baboons

> **Jargon Buster**
> social behaviour the way that two or more animals interact

- cockroaches

- bees

Other animals form complex social hierarchies. This means that the position of an animal is not a simple ranking amongst the group. Instead, for example:

- animal A might be dominant over animal B;

- animal B is dominant over animal C;

- but animal C is dominant over animal A.

Other even more complicated dominance relationships may be displayed amongst a group, which can have the potential for greater

Jargon Buster

linear hierarchy a simple ladder or ranking of dominance relationships between animals

complex hierarchy a non-linear set of dominance relationships between three or more animals

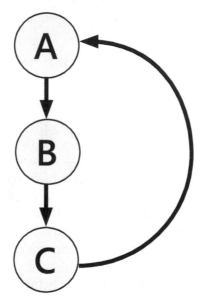

Figure 5.3 An example of a complex social hierarchy

complexity as the group gets bigger. Animals that tend to display more complex relationships include:

- cows

- horses

- dogs.

Some animals might display both linear and complex hierarchies – for instance, deer tend to be linear except for males during rutting season. Cats, meanwhile, are often solitary but can live together in social groups. The structure of those groups can be lineart or more complex – as can their relationships with other cats in the neighbourhood (see page 103).

Maintaining dominance relationships

As discussed in section 4.1, animals use different methods of communication that reinforce the dominant/submissive relationships between two animals. For instance, for dogs:

Dominant dog communication	Submissive dog communication
Making direct and intense eye contact	Looking away
Baring teeth	Mouth partly or fully closed
Growling	Whimpering
Standing tall, tail up, hackles raised, ears forward	Crouched or laid down, tail down, ears down, possibly even exposing vulnerable areas such as the belly

Each species will have its own set of specific behaviours that characterise dominant and submissive behaviour. In each case the different methods of communication allow animals to assert or submit without having to resort to aggression or violence. The benefits of this for the group as a whole are that energy is conserved and potential injury is completely avoided.

> **Activity**
>
> Choose a species and research some of the typical communication methods displayed by a dominant and a submissive animal.

Agonistic behaviour

Agonistic behaviour is any behaviour that is associated with conflict between two or more animals. Whilst this may include actual fighting and aggression, the term also includes any other behaviour that may arise out of a conflict situation, including threatening behaviour and avoidance.

Jargon Buster
agonistic behaviour associated with conflict

Threat

In order to avoid violence animals who are in conflict over some resource will normally behave in a way that is meant to intimidate the other animal. One way to do this is to behave in a way that lets the other animal know that if it came to actual violence, they would get hurt. In practice this means things like:

- making themselves look bigger, both in terms of posture and fur or hair standing up on end (e.g. cats' tails become very large and fluffy when facing down a perceived threat)

- making plenty of noise to try and frighten the opponent (e.g. roaring in big cats, growling in dogs, chest beating in gorillas, bellowing in cows, the noise of a rattlesnake)

- other clear body language, such as teeth bared, adopting a ready-to-strike posture, or movements such as running directly at the opponent.

When there is a confrontation between different species, a threat display can come from the prospective prey, to tell the predator they should not try and attack.

Avoidance

One animal can choose to back down to avoid conflict and thus prevent damage to both animals. The reasons for doing so will depend on what is at stake. Typical actions include:

- pushing away

- avoiding physical contact e.g. dodging away

- retreating or running away

- submission to the other animal, when the conflict concerns some resource, in line with the social dominance relationships – although this is not an option for predator-prey interactions.

Aggression

If threatening behaviour does not cause one of the animals to back off then it is likely to escalate to further aggressive behaviour. This includes things like:

- chasing

- pushing, headbutting

- full-on aggression – exchanging blows, biting, scratching, or other behaviour relevant to that particular species.

It is quite rare that violence occurs because the cost to both animals can be very high – even the winner.

Social bonding and affiliative behaviour

Affiliative behaviour is that which serves to develop the social bonds between two or more members of a social group. Such behaviour includes things like:

- allogrooming

- play

- group sleeping

- other forms of non-aggressive touching.

> **Jargon Buster**
> affiliative behaviour that encourages and develops social bonds

Building or reinforcing social bonds is of benefit to all animals involved, as it makes future cooperation more likely and reduces the likelihood of agonistic behaviour that leads to aggression. Therefore affiliative behaviour is mutually beneficial.

Altruism

The biological definition of altruism, or altruistic behaviour, is when an animal's action reduces its own likelihood of reproductive success whilst increasing the likelihood of another animal's reproductive success. (This definition is slightly different to the common definition of altruism which is when one organism consciously helps another for purely selfless reasons.)

Some examples of biological atruism in animals are:

- Bee colonies includes worker bees who do not reproduce but instead find food for the colony, look after the queen and guard the hive. There is no individual reproductive benefit to each worker bee for this behaviour.

- Vervet monkeys will sound an alarm to alert the social group when a predator approaches, thus potentially endangering themselves rather than keeping quiet and hiding.

Altruistic behaviour appears to be difficult to understand within the context of Darwinian theory and Darwin recognised this problem. One explanation that is widely accepted is called kin selection. It states that altruistic behaviour in a given population began in a selective way, only for close family members. This means that animals that are more likely to have the genes responsible for altruism (i.e. the close relatives) benefit from the original animal's behaviour, which gives them a reproductive advantage over other animals in the population. Thus in the next generation more animals are likely to have that gene, and so on.

> **Jargon Buster**
> altruism in biological terms, behaviour which reduces an animal's reproductive chances in favour of another animal

Quiz Questions

1 What is a) a linear hierarchy, b) complex hierarchy?

2 Give two examples of communication methods that help maintain dominance relationships.

3 What is agonistic behaviour and what are the three main types?

4 How is agonistic behaviour useful for social relationships?

5 What is affiliative behaviour? Give two examples.

6 What is the biological definition of altruism?

4.3 Mating and parent-offspring behaviour

In this topic you will learn about mating systems and strategies:

- polygamy

- monogamy

- non-associative

- courtship.

You will also learn about parental behaviour and strategies:

- bi-parental

- intensive

- no parental investment

- parent-offspring bonding

- imprinting.

Mating systems and strategies

Reproduction is at the heart of Darwin's theory of evolution. Animals have adopted different strategies for successful mating that allows them to pass on their genetic material to the next generation.

Polygamy

This is when an animal (male or female) has more than one mate of the opposite sex, but those mates are exclusive within some social group. Polygamy can be in the form of:

a) one male with multiple females (e.g. gorillas, tigers), known as polygyny

b) one female with multiple males (e.g. marmosets, tortoises), known as polyandry

c) multiple males and females in groups (e.g. chimpanzees), known as polygynandry.

The benefits of polygamy are:

- the male (a) and the female (b) increase their likelihood of reproductive success, with multiple offspring carrying their genes there is a greater likelihood that some will survive and thrive.

- the benefit for the females (a) and males (b) are in terms of resources that are controlled by the sex with multiple mates, e.g. if the females of the species in b) control territory and food then the males will need to rely on the females.

- males and females benefit in b) and c) because there is reduced competition between males (leading to less chance of injury), less chance of jealous males killing another male's offspring

- in c) there is a greater spread of genetic material across offspring which benefits all parties.

Monogamy

This is when a male and female animal form an exclusive mating relationship. It is common in birds but much less so in other animals. The benefits of monogamy are:

- shared caring of the young, with an increased likelihood of their survival and therefore of the parents' genetic material

- the burden of acquisition of resources such as food and materials for shelter are also shared.

Non-associative

This is when an animal mates indiscriminately with any number of animals from the opposite sex. This normally occurs when there is no advantage to choosing a mate, which might be because it is unclear which traits are advantageous in the environment. Examples of promiscuous animals inlcude bonobos.

Courtship

Animals that select partners do so based on factors that they perceive will give their offspring the best chance of thriving and eventually reproduce themselves. The factors depend on the species and environment in which the animals have evolved. When finding a mate, animals will often try and show their prospective partner that they do indeed posses qualities that will make them the best mate. They do this through courtship rituals. These can be in the form of:

- dances – these are ritualised movements, sometimes very complex, that an animal uses to woo a partner e.g. albatross – see https://tinyurl.com/y2ut2g2k

- a visual display to impress the prospective partner e.g. a peacock displaying his colourful tail – see https://tinyurl.com/yd29fzlp

- building objects or collecting items as part of a display – possibly to demonstrate the ability to build a nest e.g. bower birds – see https://tinyurl.com/yddaz9n9

- sounds or calling e.g. sloths – see https://tinyurl.com/pvzbfpk

- demonstrating strength or aggression e.g. silverback gorillas – see https://tinyurl.com/y2p3kapg

More often than not it is males who try and court females.

Parental behaviour and strategies

At a fundamental level, the strategies that animals use to care for their young depend on the evolutionary costs and benefits of doing so. There is a high reproductive cost for parents to look after their young – time spent looking after their young is time that animals are not spending on further reproductive activities, and finding food for the young is at the expense of their own diet. So, it is not too surprising that a great many species simply do not look after their young at all.

Parental care behaviour tend to be more complex in mammals and birds because their newborn young are often born helpless and unable to look after themselves. This means they require their parents to provide them with food, shelter and protection from predators. Because of this, there would be an even greater reproductive cost to such animals if they didn't look after their young as they would die and their genetic material would not be passed on. In more complex species, the period of care can last for a long time and also include teaching skills like hunting.

Biparental

This is when both male and female parents look after their offspring together. This is common in birds because they do not produce their own milk, and constantly finding food is very time consuming. Sharing this task across both parents results in a greater likelihood of survival for the offspring. A good example of this strategy working in practice is with emperor penguins – the hostile conditions in Antarctica means that any other parenting strategy would result in the death of the young.

Intensive

Where there is parental care, it is more common in mammals for just one parent to look after the young. Because there is a high cost to parenting, from an evolutionary point of view it makes sense that if one parent can raise the young without putting the offspring at risk then the other parent does not need to be involved. This allows the abandoning parent to pursue further reproduction.

It is normally the case that it is the male that leaves the female to care for the young by herself. This might be due to a higher reproductive cost for males than females, in that they would miss more opportunities to reproduce than females if the roles were reversed. In the case of mammals the physiological factor – i.e. the female provides milk – means that an absent male has far less impact on the likelihood of survival than an absent female.

No parental investment

Many reptiles and fish provide no care at all to their young. For instance, most snakes that lay eggs are not even present when the eggs hatch, and so the young are on their own from the first day.

Parent-offspring bonding

Species that care for their young have developed, through evolution, bonding mechanisms between parents and their children. This works in two ways:

- The parent has a strong instinct to look after its own young – it is not indifferent towards them and does not see them as a threat.

- The newborn and young completely trust their parent(s), follow them and in some cases learn from them. They have an instinct to be protected by them.

The bond normally forms at a very young age, in a certain crucial period in the offspring's life. Without such bonding the social structures and behaviours covered in this unit would not have been able to develop.

Imprinting

Filial imprinting is that between a parent and its offspring. In some species there is a hard-wired instinct to acquire some new behaviour through an external stimulus. For instance, newborn geese have an instinct to imprint onto any moving object. Normally that would be their mother but it is quite possible instead for goslings to imprint onto humans or even inanimate objects. When this happens this leads to them following humans around just as they normally would with their mother.

> **Jargon Buster**
> filial offspring

Sexual imprinting is when the young learn what to look for in a mate and again happens at a very young age. If an animal spends time with a different species when very young they can imprint upon the wrong species and try and choose them as a mate later in life. Studies show, for instance, that choice of mate in male zebra finches is strongly influenced by the animals they grew up with.

Quiz Questions

1 What is polygamy?

2 What is monogamy?

3 What does non-associative mating mean?

4 Give two examples of courtship routines.

5 What are the pros and cons of biparental and intensive parenting?

6 Why would some animals have a strategy for no parental input at all?

7 Why do some animals develop a bond between parents and offspring?

8 Explain what filial and sexual imprinting is.

END OF UNIT QUESTIONS

1. a) List **three** typical behaviours that a dog might demonstrate.   (3 marks)

_____

_____

b) List **three** atypical behaviours that a dog might demonstrate.   (3 marks)

_____

_____

2. State **three** ways in which animals benefit from grooming.

_____ (3 marks)

_____

_____

3. Describe how a cat might demonstrate territorial behaviour.   (4 marks)

_____

_____

_____

4. State **three** reasons why an animal in a zoo might display   (3 marks)
stereotypic behaviour.

_____

_____

_____

5. Explain **four** ways in which the behaviour of a domestic dog   (4 marks)
differs from that of a wolf.

_____

_____

_____

6. Explain how the environment can impact an animal's   (2 marks)
behaviour.

_____

_____

7. Explain what is meant by heredity of behaviour.   (3 marks)

_____

_____

_____

8. a) Define what is meant by instinctive behaviour.   (1 mark)

_____

b) Give **one** example of instinctive behaviour..   (1 mark)

_____

9. Describe how testosterone can influence an animal's   (1 mark)
behaviour

_____

                                                              (2 marks)
10. Describe and give an example of each of the following
communication methods.

a) Vision

_____

b) Smell

_____

                                                              (1 mark)
11. Explain the meaning of the term linear social hierarchy.

_____

12.Two dogs meet each other for the first time. Describe and
give examples of the different ways in which they might display (6 marks)
agonistic behaviour.

_____

_____

_____

_____

Preparing for your exam

The 031/531 exam has 60 marks and will last for two hours. There are around 12-15 short answer questions, worth 48 marks, split fairly equally between all three units. The final 12 marks are allocated to an Extended Response Question (ERQ), which is based on a short scenario. The ERQ requires you to draw together what you have learned in all three units and then apply it to the scenario and justify your reasoning.

The exam is designed so you can show the examiner that you can:

- recall knowledge about all of the topics in this book

- understand ideas and concepts

- apply your knowledge and understanding.

These are called **assessment objectives**. Different questions, or parts of questions, will test these different assessment objectives. Short answer questions will test the first two assessment objectives, but most of the available marks are for the second assessment objective, **understand ideas and objectives**. This means that most short answer questions will require you to show that you understand topics, and not just list or state what you know.

Short answer questions

These questions will have different forms but all of them will use certain **command verbs** in the questions. These command verbs have very specific meanings – different verbs are asking for different things. Understanding the command verbs is an important part of your preparation for the exam as they tell you what the examiner is looking for.

When a question wants you to recall knowledge, it will use command verbs like **list**, **state**, **name** etc. It will also tell you how many things you need to list, state, name. You do not need to write long answers for these questions.

When a question wants you to show your understanding – and many will – it will use words like **evaluate**, **describe**, **explain**, **summarise** etc. Words like this tell you that you need to do more than simply list things you know about the topic. If you only list what you know, or even worse use one-word answers, then you will lose marks on these questions.

Your lecturer will be able to show you a full list of command verbs that could be used in the exam, and what they mean. As part of your preparation for the exam **you should make sure you know all of the command verbs and fully understand what each one is asking you to do.**

The number of marks for each question is indicated in brackets. This number gives you a clue as to how much information you need to put down. For instance, if a question asks you to 'Compare the behaviour of an animal in the wild and in captivity', and is worth three marks, then you would need to compare three different behaviours. If you listed six behaviours then you would have wasted some precious time in the exam, because you can only receive a maximum of three marks.

Single word answers, short sentences and bullet points are all acceptable for the short answer questions - as long as they do answer the question. In fact answering in this way can save time that you can then spend on the extended response question.

Extended response question

The ERQ tests the other assessment objective: whether you can **apply your knowledge and understanding**. The ERQ is in the form of a short scenario which is designed so you can bring together knowledge from across all three units. If you do not cover some topics from all three units in your answer then you will lose marks.

The answer to the extended response question should be in the form of a short essay, written in full sentences. Spelling and grammar are not marked but are important so the examiner can understand what points you are making.

Before beginning writing an answer to the ERQ you should:

- Carefully re-read the question and identify the important words that your answer must account for.

- Take a few minutes to write a plan for your answer. This will help you to think about all of the topics you will need to cover and provide you with a structure from which you can write your full answer.

As an example, a question might ask something like:

A malnourished and pregnant cat is brought into the animal welfare centre where you work. Outline and justify how you would care for the animal.

First, you should identify the important words:

A malnourished and pregnant cat is brought into the animal welfare centre where you work. Outline and justify how you would care for the animal.

'Outline' and 'Justify' are the command verbs which your answer needs to address. If you do not justify your ideas then you cannot get the highest marks. Justify means 'explain why'.

There are a number of things you would outline in the care plan for any animal brought into the centre. But there are some specific things that you would need to think about for an animal that is 'malnourished', an animal that is 'pregnant' and for 'cats'. As well as the more general points, you need to consider the very specific needs of this particular animal. You will lose marks if you do not. You should also consider that there are other animals present in an 'animal welfare centre'.

Now you have a clear understanding of what the question is asking, you can create a plan for your answer. First, you might want to list the different topics that are relevant, for instance:

- health – routine checks, indicators of health, legislation that you will need to follow

- diseases – signs and treatment of common diseases, preventative care (for the cat and the other animals), nutritional deficiencies

- feeding requirements, feeding plan and record keeping, informed by knowledge of nutritional components of food, and the roles and functions of those nutrients

- behaviour of the animal – natural and atypical, what observed behaviours might indicate

- social behaviour – interactions with other animals, housing.

This list of topics should be drawn from all three units. If you miss topics from one unit, or they are covered in less detail than other units, you will lose marks.

Then you might want to plan out a logical structure for your answer, to feed these different topics in as appropriate. For instance, you could think about what you would need to do:

- as soon as the animal arrived

- in the first couple of hours

- during the first day

- in the first week

- over the following month.

You could work though this in order, explain in detail what you suggest and then justify why in each case. Remember to link all of your points back to the very specific scenario of this 'malnourished, pregnant cat' in the question.

Whilst the topics in each unit have been presented separately, many of them are interrelated and the ERQ wants you to show that you understand this. For instance the health of the cat in question has been affected by its poor diet, so a longer term improvement in its health may be down to the feeding plan. Its poor diet may be a sign of neglect, which in turn may have led to atypical behavioural issues. And so on.

General tips when sitting the exam

- It is a good idea to spend the first couple of minutes of the exam reading through the whole paper before attempting to answer any questions.

- A common mistake is not to read questions properly. Do not rush – make sure you understand exactly what the question is asking before attempting it.

- Identify the command verbs in each question and take a moment to recall what that verb is asking you to do.

- You should focus on answering what the question asks. Do not waste time by repeating information or writing long-winded answers that do not make any relevant points.

- If you can't answer a question don't panic. Leave it and come back to it later.

- Use the number of marks for each question as a guide for how much time you should spend on each question.

- The ERQ is worth 20% of the total marks and you should make sure you leave enough time to tackle it. Although it is the last question you do not need to leave it until last - you could consider tackling it before then. If so you should allocate a certain amount of time to focus on the ERQ, so that you have time to go back to the other questions.

- Attempt every question, even if you are not sure you know the answer!

The examination can cover topics from any of the learning outcomes in any of the units in this book. So you must ensure you have are familiar with all of those topics, and are familiar with the meaning and spelling all of the technical and specialist terms that are used throughout. This is not something you can do a few nights before the exam - so make sure you plan your revision schedule far in advance of the exam and spend plenty of time revisiting all of the content.

Index

Printed in the USA
CPSIA information can be obtained
at www.ICGtesting.com
LVHW062234240324
775357LV00036B/508

9 780992 900229